the healing garden

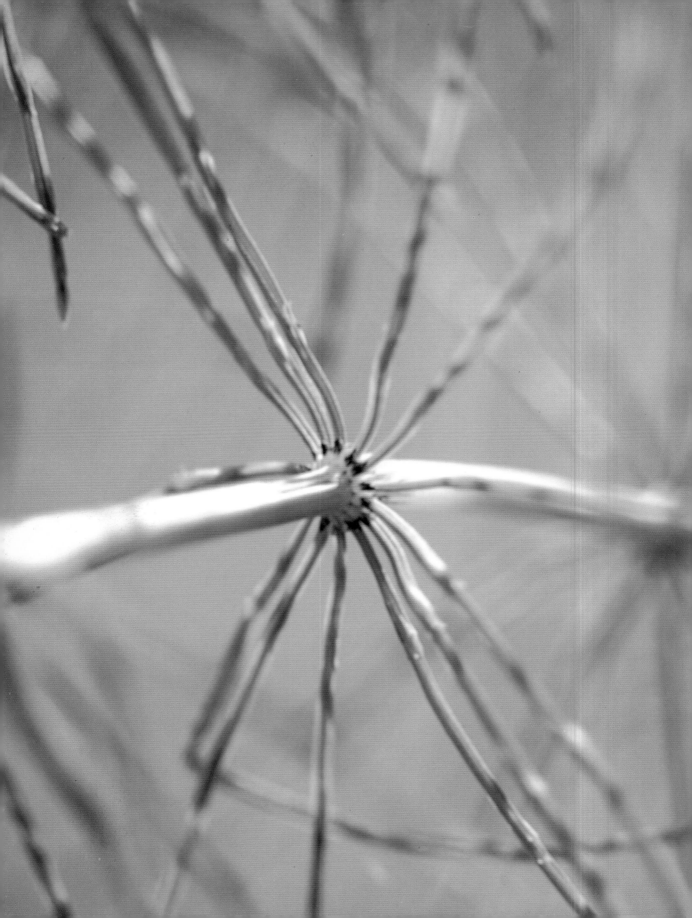

the healing garden

nature's remedies & cures

Helen Farmer-Knowles

photography by Deni Bown

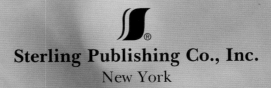

Sterling Publishing Co., Inc.

New York

A GAIA ORIGINAL

Books from Gaia celebrate the vision of Gaia, the
self-sustaining living Earth, and seek to help its readers live in
greater personal and planetary harmony.

Editor	Clare Stewart
Design	Matt Moate
Development Design	Patrick Furse
Photography	Deni Bown
Managing Editor	Pip Morgan
Production	Lyn Kirby
Direction	Patrick Nugent

Library of Congress
Cataloging-in-Publication Data available

10 9 8 7 6 5 4 3 2 1

Published in 1998 by Sterling Publishing Company, Inc
387 Park Avenue South, New York, N. Y. 10016

Originally published in Great Britain in 1998 by Gaia Books

Copyright © 1998 Gaia Books Limited, London
Text Copyright © 1998 by Helen Farmer-Knowles

Distributed in Canada by Sterling Publishing
c/o Canadian Manda Group, One Atlantic Avenue Suite 105
Toronto, Ontario, Canada M6K 3E7

Printed and bound in Italy by LEGO SpA

ISBN 0-8069-1773-3

To the reader

The Garden Healer makes no pretence to be a complete herbal, rather it is carrying on the practical tradition of a "horti-medical chest", using whatever is seasonably available.

This book is not intended for prescribing medicines, nor for curing afflictions. It is intended as a reference source on medicinal plants which are used in herbalism by qualified practitioners. Do not attempt self-diagnosis or self-treatment for any serious illness without consulting a qualified medical herbalist or doctor. Do not exceed any recommended dosages. Always consult a professional if symptoms persist. If taking prescribed medicines, seek professional advice before using herbal remedies. Never take essential oils internally. The contraindications for the use of herbs in pregnancy apply only to those used medicinally. It is perfectly safe to use herbs normally employed in cooking for culinary purposes.

Do not collect wild or cultivated herbs growing near roadsides or other sources of pollution. Cultivated herbs are better grown organically to avoid chemical contamination. Take care to correctly identify plants and do not pick restricted species.

Wherever a warning is required a symbol appears on the page. The key of warning symbols below explains the meaning of each symbol. The symbols refer you to the plant cautions at the back of the book (see pp.132-3). Do not take any herb without first checking for the warning symbols on the relevant page.

☀	General warning
✲	Avoid in pregnancy
✸	Avoid if allergic or skin sensitive
✵	Must be diagnosed/treated by professional medical doctor
✳	Do not use for children
✽	Contraindicated if you have a complaint or are on medication

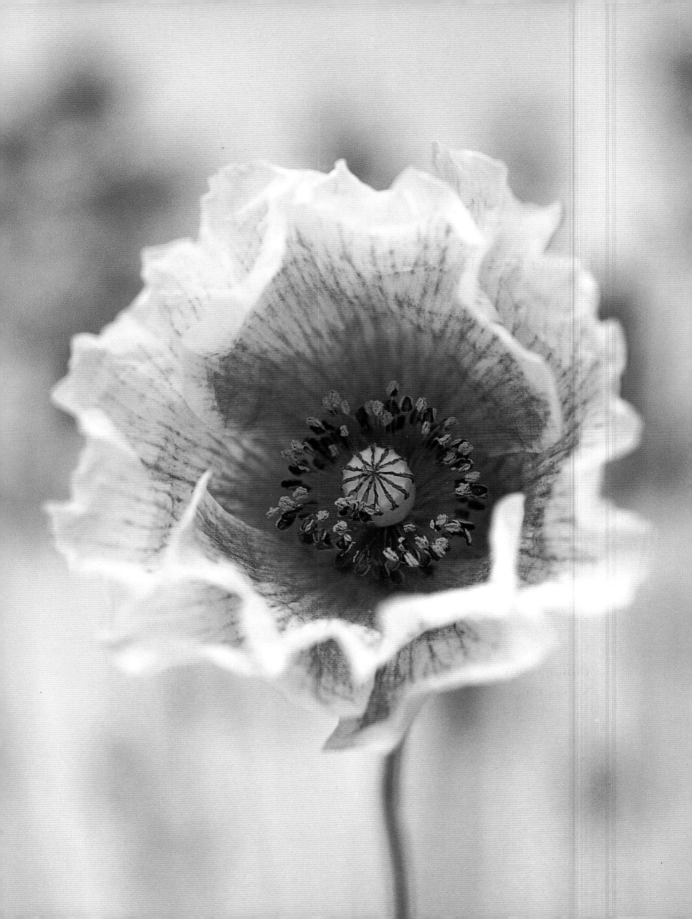

Contents

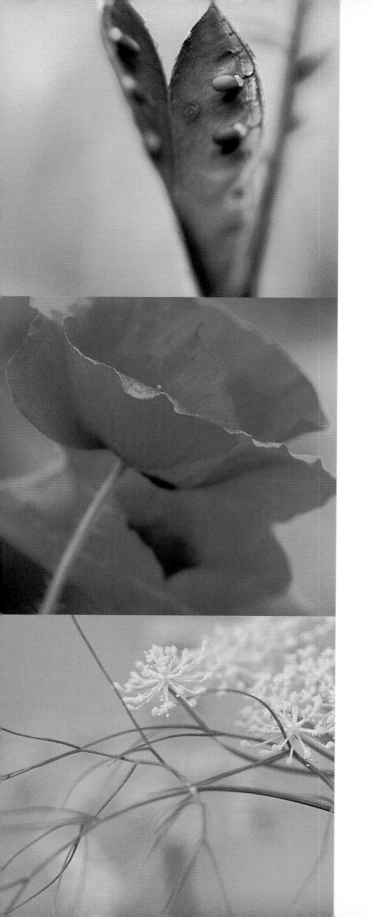

Foreword

During the course of my research into natural health and beauty I read many reference and self-help books from around the world, but it is rare to come across one so comprehensive in its contents and so sensitively written.

As an acclaimed aromatherapist, counsellor and healer, Helen Farmer-Knowles recognizes the fundamental link between our health and our beauty. In *The Garden Healer*, she combines a holistic attitude to health with a better understanding of the natural world around us. Inner vigour is the only way to achieve an outer glow of vitality, and we can all give nature a helping hand by using well-chosen botanical ingredients. We need to understand how nature can work with us to encourage our wellbeing – this book provides the key.

What I especially love about *The Garden Healer* are the many good ideas for health and beauty. From recipes for age-defying skin lotions to helpful remedies for everyday ailments that are literally good enough to eat. It's an engrossing read, being both easy to follow and full of information, including sensible safety advice. Helen Farmer-Knowles brings a new understanding to the potent healing powers of nature and shows how we can all benefit from their application to modern life.

The Garden Healer is a book for families to treasure and keep close to hand.

Liz Earle
Award-winning health & beauty author & broadcaster

Introduction

In the first book of Moses, written some 4,000 years before the birth of Christ, the building of the temple of the Sphinx and Cheops' great pyramid, we are told how the Lord God planted the Garden of Eden. This provision of the Almighty was gifted to humans to enhance their world and enjoy. Even after the Fall from grace, gardens have ever been a source of inspiration and creativity, and imbued with a spirit of adventure. From lofty trees and the rainbow spectrum of the flower border to versatile wonderful weeds, we too can savour the fruits of our labours and unlock the secrets of the healing powers sealed into every plant of Providence.

Living in the age of nuclear and computer technology often culls us from our roots. In recent times there has developed a schism between humans and the earth itself that needs to be healed. To be a Garden Healer is a simple vocation that anyone can aspire to, and, in reality as we shall see, the garden itself is the greatest healer of all.

Long before the instigation of sophisticated laboratory research and techniques, botany and medicine were two strands of the same rope. Although our forebears knew little of chemistry or pharmacology, let alone physics, throughout the development of human civilization the relationship between people, the elements, the animal kingdom and ambient vegetation has been intimate and vital.

It is no coincidence that remains of flowers have been found at the burial grounds of Neanderthal man. This was an early species that inhabited Europe for some 230,000 years, who vanished 30,000 years ago, and was first identified in the Neander Valley, near Düsseldorf, Germany, in 1856. Even these primitive people ritualized death, marked by

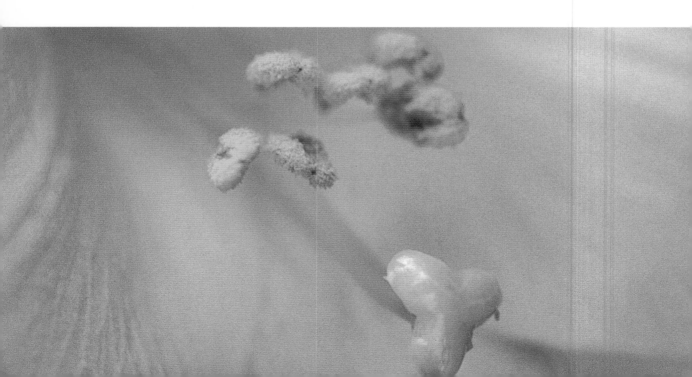

flowers set around their graves by the rest of their social group. Life was tough for our early ancestors, who were as nomadic as the wild animals of the mountains and forests, birds of the sky and fish of the rivers and seas. Being totally dependent upon their planetary environment, humans relied a great deal upon hands-on experiment and experience, and made careful selections through observation.

ANIMALS KNOW THE BEST REMEDIES

In every culture and corner of the globe people gained inestimable knowledge concerning the medicinal actions of plants through investigation of animals. Among which they observed that cats kill birds, employing the quills of their feathers to massage fur-balls up their throats; cats and dogs naturally cure their stomach upsets by eating grasses; sick sheep automatically look for yarrow to eat; wild boar poisoned by henbane use the roots of the carline thistle as an antidote. Horses eat the young fresh dandelions of spring to purify their blood and bears come out of hibernation in search of "bear's garlic" to help cleanse their system.

The birds of the air and the beasts of the field all know the best herbal remedy for what ails them. Humans were not perhaps at first so intuitive, but had this lead of natural animal testing to aid them and gradually learned to use nature's healing powers for themselves. Historically, colours, shapes, forms and the scent of plants influenced their choice. Examples of this are mandrake, shaped like a human; the heart-shaped leaves of the violet and the pulmonary patterns of lungwort. Still today many herbs are used in their crude form, and all over the world various flowers, leaves, roots and seeds are chewed for their numerous beneficial properties.

NATURE'S LARDER

It was not only plants' curative properties that assisted people's health, or plant forms of proteins and some fats, but the vital vitamins and mineral salts contained therein as nourishment in the form of food. Nature's larder has been interfered with and depleted in essence through humankind's interventions and resultant pollutions. This partly stems from supporting a vastly over-populated world, as much as from detractions and unnatural innovations in the realms of agriculture and horticulture.

Organic food itself can form the best barrier of preventive medicine for the immune system. Many plants that are herbs can be grown for their value as preventive medicine, as well as remedial medicine. In accordance with climate and geographical location, we can add them to our garden's healing capacity, whether designated as herb or weed.

THE DEVELOPMENT OF MEDICINE

Archaeology has proved, and recorded history has chronicled from Ancient China and Egypt onwards, that the early tools and methods of physicians and surgeons were very crude. Medicine was "natural" until the time of Jenner's discovery of vaccination in 1796, then Pasteur's of micro-organisms and pasteurization. When J. C. Tiemann, the eminent German nineteenth-century chemist, isolated ionone in 1893 he initiated the era of synthetic perfumes. Unwittingly, he also sparked a firestorm in the production of synthetic drugs, with little notion of their side-effects. This in turn helped to fuel a radical change in the approach of the medical profession, which became centred on science.

Throughout history people have healed themselves with plants. Both the Egyptians and the biblical Babylonians were keen gardeners.

The mythological Greeks continued this healing tradition making prolific use of plants in their medicine. Later in history medical knowledge lay in the hands of the Celtic Druids. Come the Middle Ages, medicine and the healers of the world were either to be found in the gardens of the local folk herbalists known as Wise Women, or in the Christianized locations of abbey and monastery gardens.

THE COTTAGE GARDEN
In Britain during the Industrial Revolution, in cities where the poor could not afford a doctor, lack of lore and expediency caused the use of gin, or "Mother's Ruin," to dull pain. In order to have access to healing plants the workers cultivated their own source by developing the cottage garden with all its healing qualities.

Tear humans away from their natural habitat and they are disconnected from the soil that sustains them through life and welcomes them in death. The rapid growth of industry in Victorian Britain forced the rural population into cities. Rather than lose their healing heritage, they took with them the earth and plants from their gardens and cultivated potted plants in their city abodes. Today's city dwellers have to be grateful to these pioneers. It is they, with their seven sacred plants (the "Florists' Flowers") – anemone, auricula, carnation, hyacinth, pinks, polyanthus and ranunculus – who showed the way to our indoor gardening. This became elevated from windowsill to window boxes and patios of the cities where we now happily grow culinary and remedial herbs.

In a stressed modern era everyone, wherever possible, can lighten the load and help give breath to the lungs of the world. Plants feed our needs far beyond replenishment of all-important oxygen. The Garden Healer has a unique opportunity to assail the

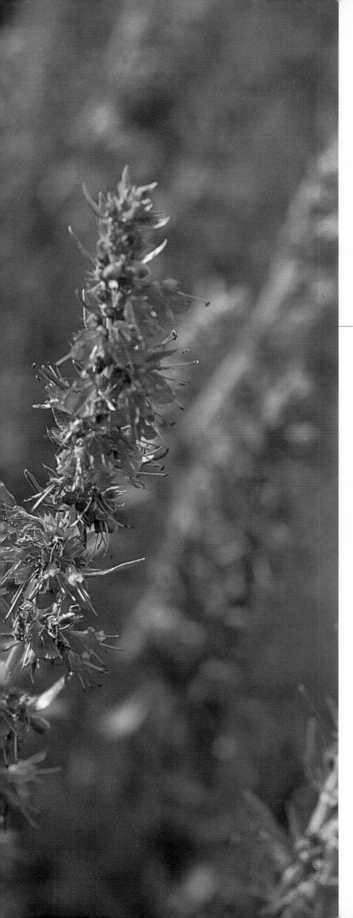

senses with delights. Whilst a blind person is deprived of the sight of beautiful flowers, he or she can at least appreciate their texture and scent, and gain solace from a garden in which the sound of water is balm to the spirits. In a garden the deaf too can experience a musical symphony of colour and scent. It is, therefore, important for the city-dweller to grow plants that are not only remedial but colourful and fragrant, and able to soothe the senses cut off from nature in the physically invasive ferro-concrete jungle.

OUR SENSE OF SMELL

Medicinal remedies and recipes are invaluable, but there is one primary sense that can aid us all – smell. Our sense of smell has somewhat diminished since we were hunter-gatherers, but the old brain, the limbic system, which interprets smell, still forms first in any foetus. Aromatic plants and flowers are tools that may be used in the garden to calm the nerves, de-stress the mind, restore the body and salve the soul. Fragrance appeals to our psyche, which means spirit – any invalid or convalescent will benefit from not only the sight of coloured plants, but also their scent. Moreover, for those of us who cannot "dig and delve" the garden is a healer that can be planned with much to offer.

We cannot deny the enormous benefits that medicine has given us through the development of anaesthetics, antiseptic surgery, obstetrics and gynaecology. The charge is that in the rush to profit from scientific advances, the best of what had gone before in "natural medicine" was discounted, allowed to disappear, sometimes without trace, and, worst of all, not investigated or researched further until recently.

Feelings of instability have triggered a nostalgic craving for tradition and equilibrium. It is only now on this uncertain planet, inundated with the press of sheer numbers of populace and increasing degrees of pollution, that science has regenerated the desire and intelligence to examine the integrity of traditional medicine. The human soul yearns for poetry, music and romance – the beautiful, sensuous and functional garden endowed with healing power can give it back to us. As the third millennium approaches, a new renaissance dawns: a worldwide quest to find answers in nature, the most valuable inheritance of our past, which lives in our present, and gives gladly to our future health.

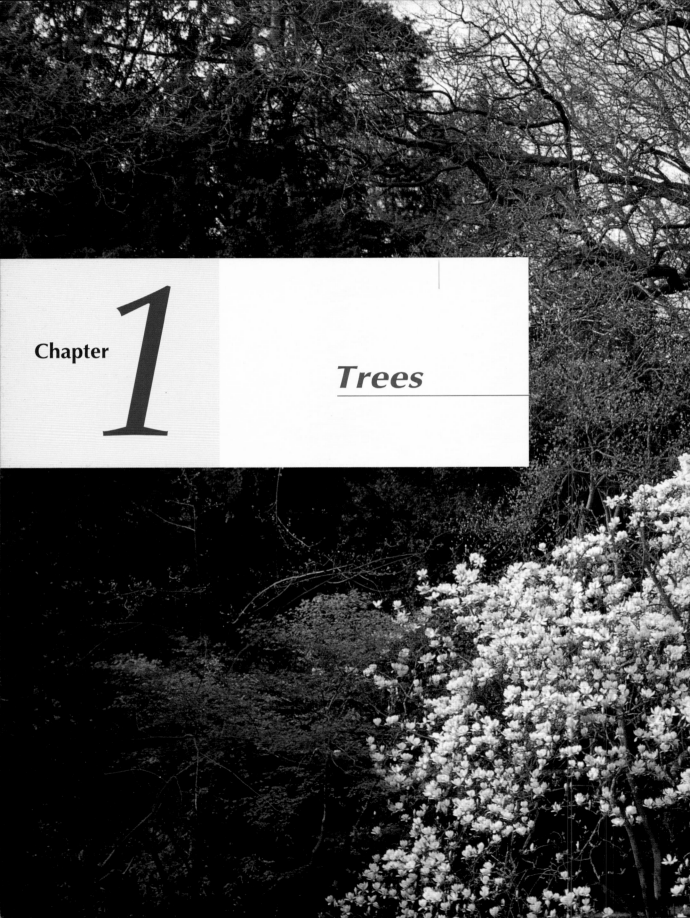

Chapter

1

Trees

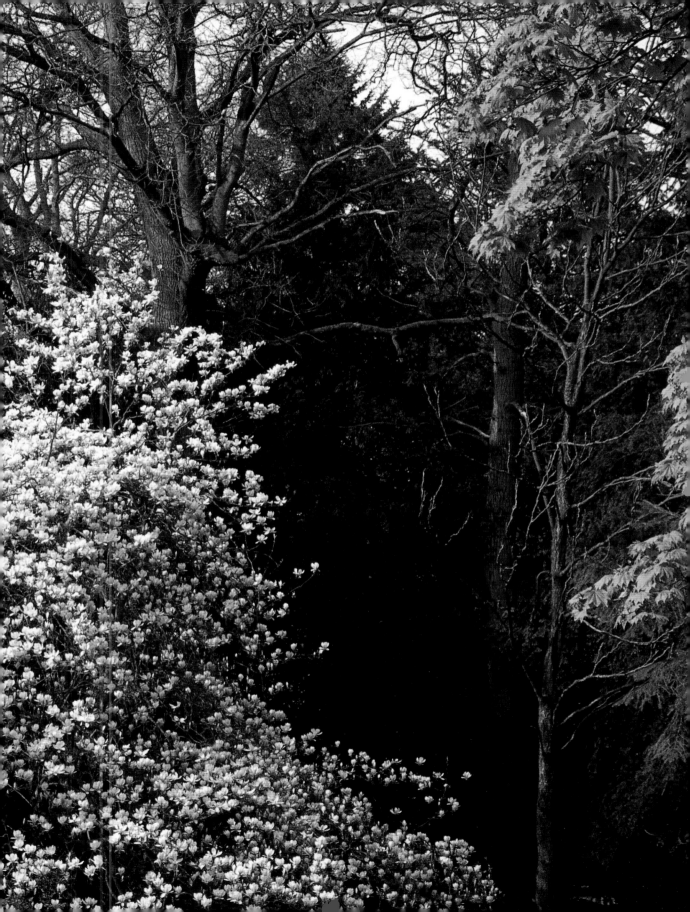

Trees

We are so fortunate to live on this particular planet with trees as our large flora. The tree-canopy is earth's protector, nature's umbrella and parasol, home to the birds and refuge for animals and once-primitive humans, as well as providing food, drink, shelter and clothing. The Bible story of creation mentions neither fragrance nor flowers. The first plants beyond aquatic single-cell organisms and algae that developed on earth are known to have been ferns and trees.

The cranium-like earth and its tectonic movement divided up our landmass into continents and countries, creating biodiversity within different climates, thus contributing to basic plant distribution. Other distributions came via the movements of birds and other animals, flotation of flotsam and jetsam in the seas and rivers, and finally by mankind's nomadic wanderings and later travel across continents.

Trees have sustained and maintained our lives globally from earliest times. First they gave us the primal element of fire, then later in Mesopotamia in 3,500 BC came the invention of the solid wooden wheel. Its very blueprint for design is described within the circles that define a tree's age and growth. In the rain-forests, trees and their leaves still provide shelter, food and medicine for Aboriginal peoples. Elsewhere they formed tools and furniture, transport and housing, derivatives and drugs, fulfilling every basic need of life.

North Americans are justly proud of the longevity of their giant redwood trees, the British rightly revere their patriarchal oak and the Mediterranean peoples venerate their ancient yews. However, it is the antipodean Aboriginal peoples who presently carry the crown for possessing the oldest tree on earth. It has been scientifically calculated that when

HORSE CHESTNUT

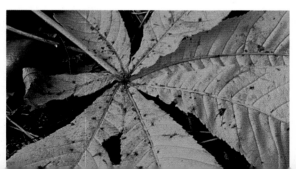

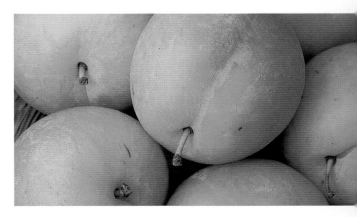

PLUMS

they first moved through the rainforest some 36,000 years ago, there existed a species, "king's holly", which was already at least 7,000 years old. We can surmise that they used this plant in their magic and medicine. Therefore, this Tasmanian find suggests that humanity's relationship with trees and their healing uses is earlier than previously believed.

TREE WORSHIP
It is well documented that, at the dawn of European history, the land was covered with immense primeval forests with oases of clearings like natural green temples. Mankind's need for worship turned naturally to trees. Trees are at the very roots of our religious worship from the Greek Arcadian oak and pines to the Celtic oak-worship of the Druids. The East gave us the Cabbalistic "Tree of Life" and every culture has its own sacred tree. The Greek wooded sanctuary of the Healing

Temple of Aesculapius, at Cos, charged 1,000 drachmas as the penalty for cutting down a cypress tree, and in the Forum of Rome, the sacred fig-tree of Romulus was glorified. Germans, Slavs, Lithuanians and Finns all worshipped trees. In the historic capital of Uppsala, in Sweden, there was a sacred grove in which every tree was regarded as divine.

Trees are far from just a practical necessity. They light our lives with love and, even if the initials, hearts and arrows incised into their bark is unwonted vandalism, they bear witness to the romance of youth. Trees have a beauty that touches all our senses, from the exotic scents of tropical frangipani (*Plumeria rubra*) to the diva (*Magnolia sprengeri*) that sheds its otherworldly April incense in a temperate arboretum. We can revel in the sight of white-blossomed blackthorn (*Prunus spinosa*) that heralds spring and delights the heart at winter's demise. And hawthorn (*Crataegus monogyna*)

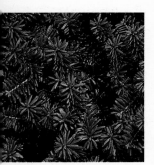

ABIES BALSAMEA

*"Except during the nine months
before he draws his first breath, no
man manages his affairs
as well as a tree does."*
**George Bernard Shaw
(1856-1950)**

announces the arcane May-tide rites of fertility. Glowing "candles" of the horsechestnut (*Aesculus hippocastanum*) give magical conkers, while sycamore (*Acer pseudoplatanus*) provides "aeroplanes" to childhood games. Trees' beauty and infinite variety of colour and bloom, together with their visual shapes, scents and sounds, speak to our spiritual dimension: they uplift us and heal us with their being in all possible ways – emotionally, mentally and physically.

HEALING TREES

The universal silver fir (*Abies alba*) relieves the ubiquitous common cold and from its leaves and resin come essential oils to alleviate rheumatism and neuralgia. The Canadian balsam fir (*Abies balsamea*) of Native American Indian prominence has seen off venereal disease in its time, is used to treat chest infections, and its antiseptic ointments and creams salve wounds and burns. Famous for food, Mediterranean people value their pine as provider of pine kernels to make Italian pesto and other culinary triumphs, and it gives shade to the delectable *Setas/ceps* (mushrooms) of Spain. In southern France, and in all parts of Europe, the sweet chestnut (*Castanea sativa*) is an astringent herb with anti-rheumatic effects. The leaves when infused can control coughing, especially whooping cough. It is a hair colourant, and provides us with delicious *marrons glacés.*

In central and southern Europe, not only the Greeks praise the bay laurel (*Laurus nobilis*), which grows in the Canary Islands and the Azores, as an aromatic stimulant herb which lends its flavour and remedial qualities to cooking. It also aids digestion and is locally antiseptic. The common elder (*Sambucus nigra*) is a veritable treasure chest of culinary, cosmetic and medicinal herbal properties. Known in Greece as "the tree of musical pipes", the elder is found growing from Europe to Western Asia and North Africa. It gives us flowers and fruits, infusions and creams that are cooling, lower fever, reduce inflammation and soothe irritation. Its leaves are insecticidal, antiseptic and healing, and its berries grace our palate as wine or jelly, alleviating rheumatic complaints.

Other fruit trees add to our daily welfare, such as the plum (*Prunus* x *domestica*), which gives vitamin E and potassium, remedying abdominal upsets, nausea and constipation. We can indulge ourselves and grow ornamentals from Japan, China and Hawaii. Romantic Japanese pepper (*Zanthoxylum piperitum*), for example, will flavour our soups and meat dishes. At the same time we know it will act upon the spleen and stomach, lowering blood pressure with bactericidal and fungicidal effects. Or we can treat ourselves to the fragrant yellow flowers of the American Oregon grape (*Mahonia*

JAPANESE PEPPER

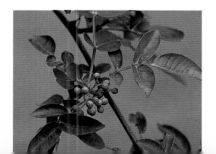

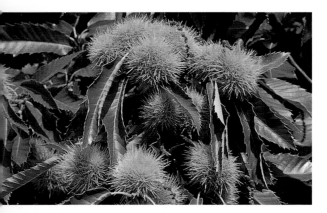

SWEET CHESTNUT

aquifolium) – its roots will stimulate the bile flow, release toxins, and can be infused to aid dry eczema, gall bladder complaints and even hepatitis B. There is no limit to the diversity and type of healing we can put into and take from the trees in our gardens.

Everyone who has some space can plant at least one small tree in their garden, even if it is only for shade, endowing it with colour and scent, a place to celebrate romance and love or honour celibate meditation. Trees are a psychological and tactile reminder of human continuity. Maybe we cannot plant trees for ourselves, only our grandchildren, but they are a precious healing inheritance we can gift to our world.

Lime or Linden Tree

Gardens have reposed in the shade of scented lime trees (*Tilia spp.*) since the Ancient Egyptians. A holy tree of the Ancient Greeks, Germans and Slavs, with the power to ward off destruction by lightning, it is believed to absorb disease when touched. The French serve tea in the afternoon beneath the calming scented silver lime (*T. tomentosum*) to calm hyper-active or fractious children.

SMALL-LEAVED LIME (TILIA CORDATA)

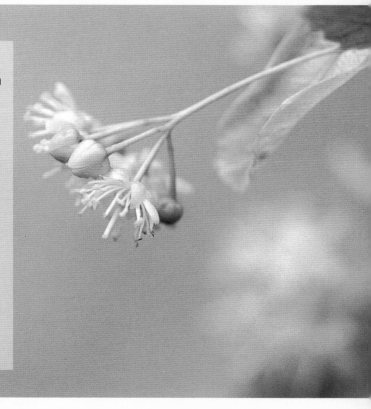

Skin Conditioning Night Cream

Melt 1 oz (25 g) beeswax in bain-marie and blend with 100 ml (4 fl oz, approx. 110 ml) cocoa butter. For stronger mixture combine 50 ml cocoa butter and 50 ml macerated sweet almond oil. Alternatively to beeswax, cocoa butter and oil, add 30 drops linden absolute (1½ %), mix in when cool before setting to avoid evaporation of its volatile constituents. Decant quickly into clean glass jars. When completely set, cover, label, date and store in a cool place.

Tip: Linden absolute may be added to ready prepared base creams, lotions and bath gels for skin-softening effect at a maximum of 1½ %, as an absolute is stronger and more concentrated than some essential oils.

Healing Uses: Infusions (see p.122) of *Tilia spp.* are used for nervous disorders; headaches, sinus in particular, catarrh; indigestion and high blood pressure. The flower blossoms are safe and easy to use. A decoction (see p.123) of limeflowers added to a base cream makes a good skin cleanser. A bath bag of blossoms is very relaxing. A hot infusion (see p.122) or tea of lindenflowers treats colds, is a relaxant for irritable children and relieves nervous exhaustion in hard-pressed adults. It also helps PMS. Mildly astringent linden absolute extracted from the dried flowers may be used in a massage (1½ %, 1 drop to 3 ml carrier oil) to similar effect: it is antispasmodic, bechic, cephalic and diaphoretic, an emollient sedative and nervine tonic.

Eucalpytus or Blue Gum

Eucalyptus, originally from Australia and an Aboriginal remedy, is a powerful antiseptic used for infections and fevers, for which it is now universally employed. Although some species of eucalyptus do not survive the winters of the Northern Hemisphere, it grows in protected micro-climates in Britain and several varieties of shrubby species do very well even in the midst of urban environments.

Healing Uses: The essential oil has analgesic, anti-neuralgic, anti-rheumatic, anti-spasmodic, antiviral and bactericidal properties among others. *E. dives* will destroy *staphylococci* present on the skin. The broad-shaped leaves or oil of the Australian peppermint species, *E. dives*, are used externally as an anti-inflammatory antiseptic, for bronchitis, mouth and throat infections, influenza and colds, sciatica, arthritis and sprains. It makes an aromatic stimulant and good decongestant inhalation, a spasm relaxant for coughs, and is excellent for expectoration. It also lowers fevers in influenza and colds.

Home Uses: To relieve the pain of sprains, use the warming and slightly anaesthetic effect of diluted essential oil in a base oil or ointment (see p.125) or make from plant material.

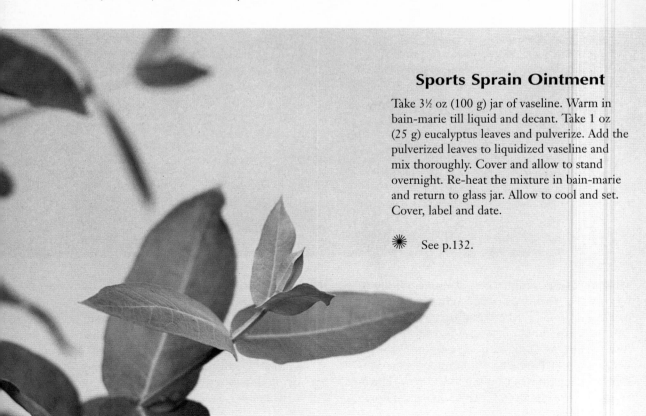

Sports Sprain Ointment

Take 3½ oz (100 g) jar of vaseline. Warm in bain-marie till liquid and decant. Take 1 oz (25 g) eucalyptus leaves and pulverize. Add the pulverized leaves to liquidized vaseline and mix thoroughly. Cover and allow to stand overnight. Re-heat the mixture in bain-marie and return to glass jar. Allow to cool and set. Cover, label and date.

✳ See p.132.

BLUE GUM (EUCALPYTUS GLOBULUS)

Holly

The holly is a truly cosmopolitan plant, and perhaps the most ancient tree on earth. Spanning many cultures and religions, holly fetishes were practised by the Zoroasters of Persia and India as well as the classical Greeks and Romans. *Ilex paraguensis* is the maté tea of Paraguay, Brazil and Argentina. Some Native American Indians regard maté as a panacea.

COMMON HOLLY (ILEX AQUIFOLIUM)

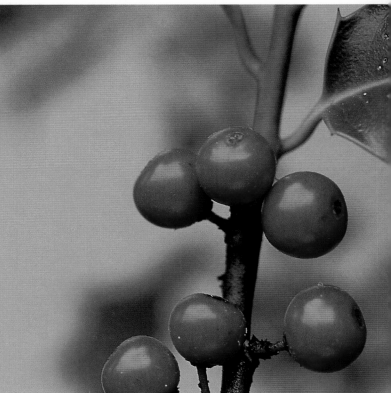

Ilex Energy Buzz

Purchase dried young *I. paraguensis* leaves. Use 1 tsp (5 ml) leaves to 1 cup spring water. Pour boiling water over leaves. Stand and cover for 10 minutes to draw or infuse.

Drink this maté tea as a specific energy booster on occasion. Use only young leaves. Maté should not be drunk with meals as tannins inhibit absorption of other nutrients. Berries are poisonous to people if eaten. Maté is an alternative to manufactured products of guarana.

None should be taken to excess, as too much caffeine will cause the heart to race and can be injurious to liver function through over-rapid release of toxins into the system.

Healing Uses: A bitter herb, American holly (*I. opaca*) is a bronchial remedy. South American maté "tea" made from the leaves of *I. paraguensis* is also grown and drunk in Spain and Portugal as "yerba maté". It is a transient energy booster due to its caffeine content. Although diuretic, it stimulates the nervous system, temporarily raising mental potency, and is slightly analgesic. It assists fatigue, headache, migraine, neuralgic and rheumatic pain, and is used to alleviate ancillary melancholy. It relaxes spasms and clears toxins, and has been used to treat diabetes. "Mao-tung-ching" (*I. rotunda* syn. *I. pubescens*) is a Chinese herbal treatment for coronary cases. Trials have shown that at least 90% of sufferers were relieved of agonizing chest pain, or it was much reduced.

Mimosa

Out of the land of Egypt, mimosa is one of a tribe of remedial acacia that grace the earth all over the globe. From Australia, silver wattle (*Acacia dealbata*) is a florist's mimosa and the national emblem. Mimosa's springtime golden coronet of violet-scented florescence is associated with the South of France. "Prickly Moses" is cultivated in the Mediterranean to produce cassie oil and has naturalized in isolation.

Healing Uses: Adaptable mimosa flourishes in niches of urban micro-climates everywhere. The sight of the blossom is so warmly uplifting, and the tree's scent is calming on the nervous system. *A. farnesiana* is an aromatic stimulant that relieves tension. The leaves contain insecticidal compounds. The flowers make sweet bags and pot-pourris and its absolute is used in perfumes.

Home Uses: Pick flowers for drying when first in bloom. Mimosa is remedial and useful to cosset skin. Its nervine and skin-softening properties can alleviate the itching and psychological discomfort of psoriasis (a skin disorder that is often hereditary, and which may be triggered by anxiety). Make up a bath bag of mimosa flowers and add to the bath water.

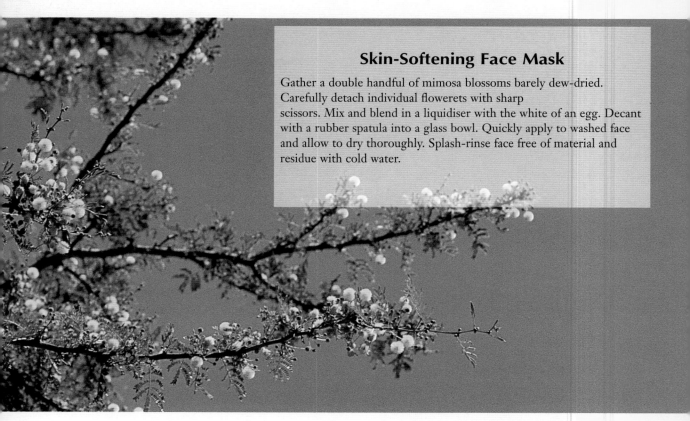

Skin-Softening Face Mask

Gather a double handful of mimosa blossoms barely dew-dried. Carefully detach individual flowerets with sharp scissors. Mix and blend in a liquidiser with the white of an egg. Decant with a rubber spatula into a glass bowl. Quickly apply to washed face and allow to dry thoroughly. Splash-rinse face free of material and residue with cold water.

PRICKLY MOSES, HUISACHE (ACACIA FARNESIANA)

Apple

Apples are profoundly rooted in British and European folklore and, like all spherical fruits, symbolic of the globe. The biblical apple *tappuah*, the Assyrian Herbal's *hashuru*, was used to treat venereal disease, later to be copied in America for gonorrhoea. Ayurvedic *tuffah*, sour apples and their pips, are eaten to strengthen the heart. Apple fragrance is associated with the breath of the dying, but its blossom signals renewal of life.

CRAB APPLE (MALUS FLORIBUNDA)

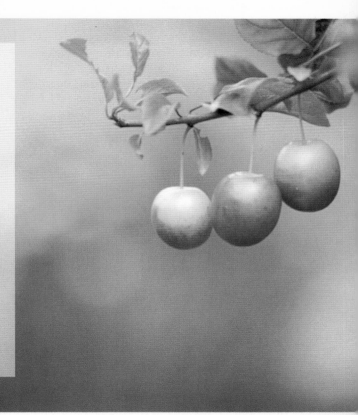

Detoxificant for Arthritis

1 tbsp (15 ml) organic cider vinegar
5 fl oz (150 ml) boiled hot water
Put vinegar in glass and pour over water. Take in morning and at night for a week. Reduce dosage in second week to once a night or morning for at least six weeks.
Tips: If arthritic, consult your doctor, as you may experience inflammation and pain when the action on the uric crystals lodged in the joints begins to work. This may occur within 2-3 days of taking the first dose. Many people experience long-term relief and reduction of symptoms when this regime is employed consistently over a long period.

Healing Uses: Apples are a good source of vitamin C, anti-oxidant and anti-toxic, helping to maintain the immune system. They are low in calories, an excellent aid for obesity, and contain a high concentration of fructose, a simple sugar sweeter than sucrose, which metabolizes slowly and assists in the balance of blood sugar levels. Ripe raw apples aid constipation and stewed treat diarrhoea and gastroenteritis. Internally apples improve skin complexion, assist acne, aid catarrh, relieve emotional stress, and help digestion, benefitting health and increasing vigour.
Home Uses: Eat "An apple a day..." for general health or drink pure juice. Use raw in salads, concentrated jelly with cold meats and desserts, organic cider vinegar in salad dressings and marinades. Grated raw apple is highly detoxificant and assists recovery in gastric poisoning.

Mountain Ash

A member of the rose family, the mountain ash, commonly called the rowan or quicken-tree, is full of mysticism. Legends of the tree abound, many telling of its magical proficiency as an antidote to witchcraft. The rowan's grace when flowering has great healing appeal to the visual sense. Its foliage unfolds in glorious crimsons and scarlets in autumn. When fruiting it displays splendid orange and ruby-red berries.

Healing Uses: Rowan berries are a renowned natural resource of vitamin C and a cure for scurvy. Infusions (see p.122) and decoctions (see p.123) of berries can be used as a gargle for sore throats and inflamed tonsils. The fumes of the burned rowan leaves are good to inhale for asthma.

Home Uses: A simple Scottish recipe for rowan jelly is a good way to use the fresh material and store it as a tonic. It makes a constitutional winter booster of vitamin C, wards off sore throats, and is practical to add to a variety of dishes.

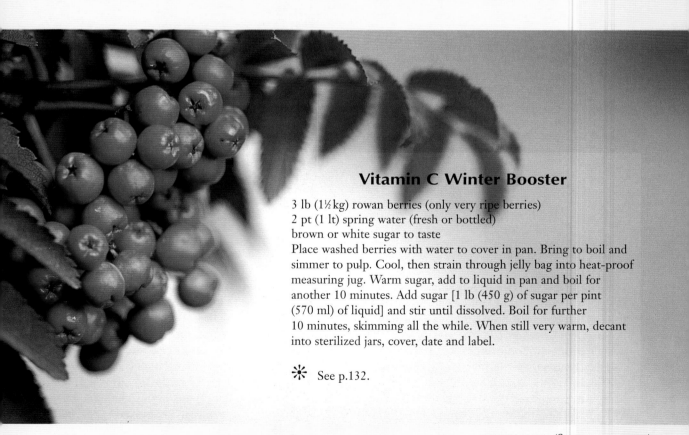

Vitamin C Winter Booster

3 lb (1½ kg) rowan berries (only very ripe berries)
2 pt (1 lt) spring water (fresh or bottled)
brown or white sugar to taste
Place washed berries with water to cover in pan. Bring to boil and simmer to pulp. Cool, then strain through jelly bag into heat-proof measuring jug. Warm sugar, add to liquid in pan and boil for another 10 minutes. Add sugar [1 lb (450 g) of sugar per pint (570 ml) of liquid] and stir until dissolved. Boil for further 10 minutes, skimming all the while. When still very warm, decant into sterilized jars, cover, date and label.

☀ See p.132.

MOUNTAIN ASH (SORBUS AUCUPARIA)

Silver Birch

Growing world-wide from North America and Britain, to the Himalayas, Western Asia, and Northern Africa, the leaves of the silver birch turn to autumn gold before shedding their bounty to the ground. The silver birch is one of our oldest providers of medicinal remedies. It remains one of the most graceful trees on earth, sweet scented when in full leaf in May, especially after spring rains.

SILVER BIRCH (BETULA PENDULA)

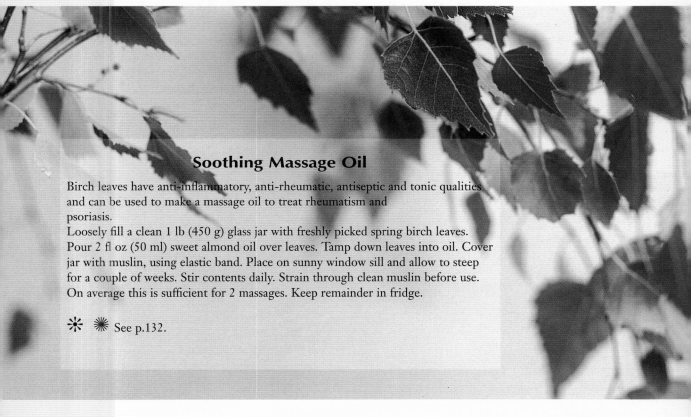

Soothing Massage Oil

Birch leaves have anti-inflammatory, anti-rheumatic, antiseptic and tonic qualities and can be used to make a massage oil to treat rheumatism and psoriasis.
Loosely fill a clean 1 lb (450 g) glass jar with freshly picked spring birch leaves. Pour 2 fl oz (50 ml) sweet almond oil over leaves. Tamp down leaves into oil. Cover jar with muslin, using elastic band. Place on sunny window sill and allow to steep for a couple of weeks. Stir contents daily. Strain through clean muslin before use. On average this is sufficient for 2 massages. Keep remainder in fridge.

✳ ✾ See p.132.

Healing Uses: Scots Celts tap spring sap for "birch blood" to treat bladder and kidneys, purify uric sediment and dissolve stones. The sap is anti-rheumatic and a remedy for gout. An infusion of birch leaf tea is used for similar effect [2 tsp (10 ml) per cup, steeped for 20 minutes. Take 1-1½ cups per day]. Apply fresh wet inner skin of bark externally to allay severe muscular pain.

Home Uses: For arthritic pain lay birch leaves in a warm bed, which induces a sweat and brings relief. Make a decoction (see p.123) of *B. alba* birch leaves to apply to any congested or irritated skin condition, and add a separate decoction to the bath.

Juniper

The West associates the juniper berry with spices and gin. The plant grows comfortably in the northern hemisphere – Canada, Scandinavia and Europe – and loves the Mediterranean and the Baltic as well as Asia. Its pungent scent, which cleanses, stimulates and revives, comes from the silvery-purple berries. These appear on the female bush only and take 3 years to ripen from green.

Healing Uses: Juniper berry, and especially its essential oil, is a great cleanser on a psychological and auric, as well as physical, level. The herb is effective for diarrhoea, convulsions, hallucinations and personality changes. Infusions (see p.122) of berries are diuretic and can treat cystitis. Do not use if infection has reached kidneys.

Home Uses: The oil may be used in moderation for oedema and cellulite. Either add 3-6 drops to the bath or use in a carrier oil for massage (1-2% maximum). Oils added to creams and ointments (see p.125) help with acne and dermatitis, oily complexions, and make a good skin toner. A massage or inhalation helps the immune system cope with secondary infections caused by colds and influenza. Employed in massage juniper berry oil is particularly useful for easing PMS.

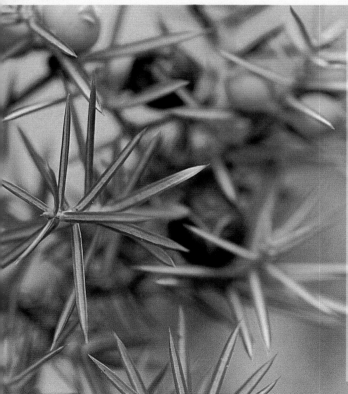

Juniper Berry Oil for PMS

Premenstrual syndrome is a condition that affects many women, causing nervousness, unwarranted irritability, and emotional disturbance prior to starting a period. Some women experience these symptoms about 10 days before menstruation. This is often accompanied by headache and/or depression. Juniper berry oil used in the bath (max. 6 drops) is ideal for healing this condition (associated with the accumulation of salt and water in the tissues), helping with any accompanying oedema.

✳ ❉ ✺ ❀ See pp.132-3.

COMMON JUNIPER (JUNIPERUS COMMUNIS)

Magnolia

Magnolia is the Adam and Eve of all trees, from which many others descended. Frequently first to brave the winter's cold, the feminine primordial shape, luxurious size and sensuous scent of magnolia's blooms, gladden the eye and inspire the soul. From Asia to America, magnolias can be found gracing the gardens of Europe or the hills of Katmandu and Japan. The Chinese medicinal *M. liliiflora* has a delicious fragrance.

LILY-FLOWERED MAGNOLIA (MAGNOLIA LILIIFLORA 'NIGRA')

Magnolia Cream

Crush into a wide-necked glass jar as many freshly fallen magnolia petals as you can. Cover with sweet almond or coconut oil (avocado for very dry skin). Seal and leave for 10-14 days in warm dark cupboard, shaking daily. Strain and decant liquid into clean jar and repeat with fresh material until liquid is scented to your satisfaction – usually three times for light-scented aromas. Strain and re-strain (single then double muslin) into clean amber/blue bottle. Add a drop of wheatgerm oil. The maceration is best added to moisturizing cream base without delay. Seal, date and label. Keep in cool dark place.

 See p.133.

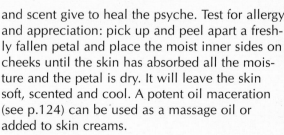
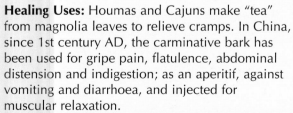

Healing Uses: Houmas and Cajuns make "tea" from magnolia leaves to relieve cramps. In China, since 1st century AD, the carminative bark has been used for gripe pain, flatulence, abdominal distension and indigestion; as an aperitif, against vomiting and diarrhoea, and injected for muscular relaxation.

Home Uses: The most important medicine of magnolia is the uplifting pleasure that its sight and scent give to heal the psyche. Test for allergy and appreciation: pick up and peel apart a freshly fallen petal and place the moist inner sides on cheeks until the skin has absorbed all the moisture and the petal is dry. It will leave the skin soft, scented and cool. A potent oil maceration (see p.124) can be used as a massage oil or added to skin creams.

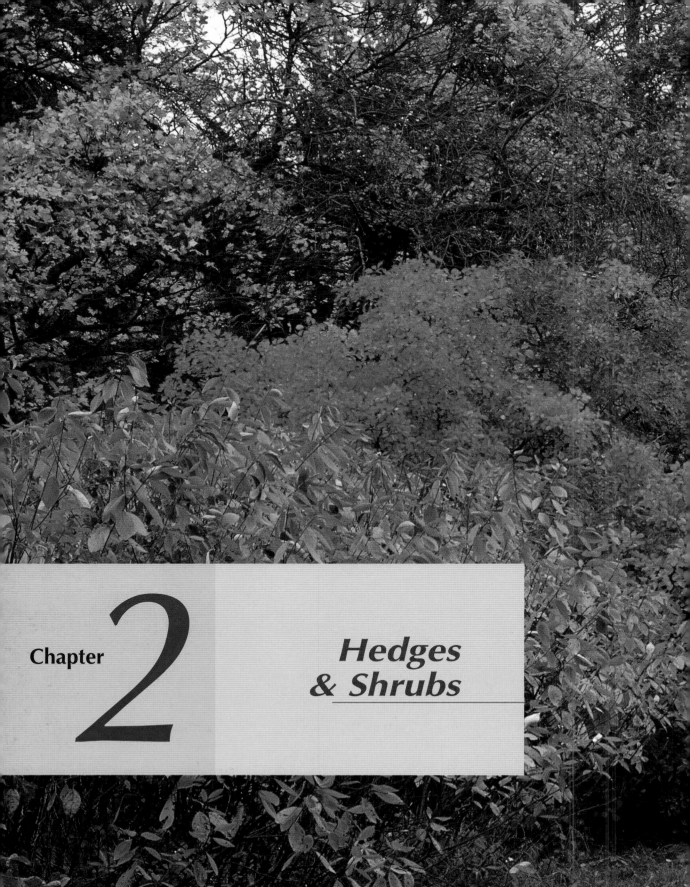

Chapter

2

Hedges & Shrubs

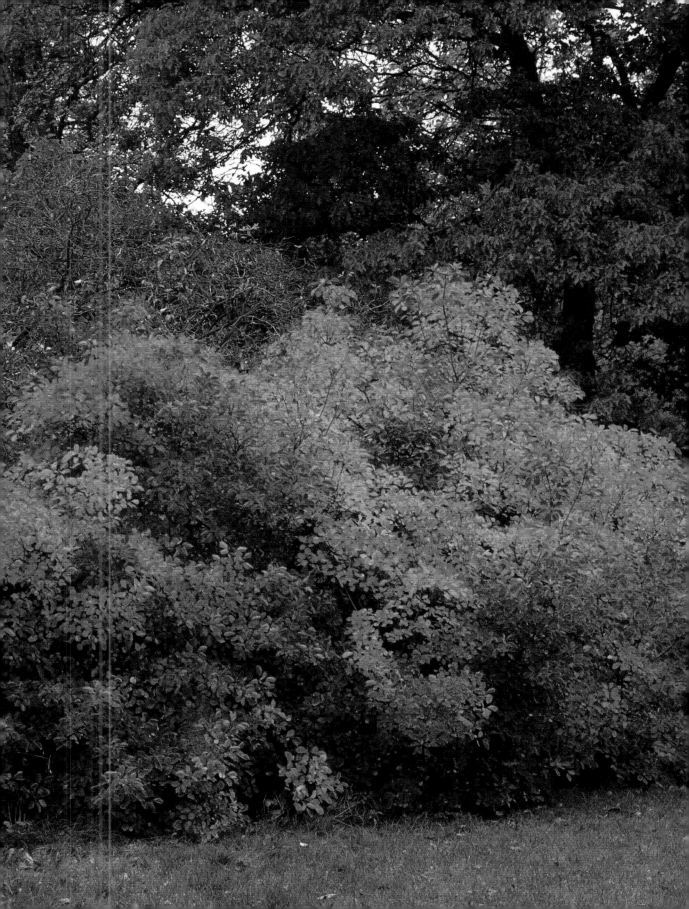

Hedges & Shrubs

The magic of the practical common-or-garden hedge abides in witchcraft. Black or white witches and enchantresses were well versed in herbalism and kept their property and gardens of mystery and magic enclosed behind hedgerows – the living garden fence. For whether in woodland or back garden their herbs were picked in secrecy. "Hedge" is, in fact, derived from the word for "hag", and hags, crones or witches were believed to shelter in hedges, particularly the hawthorn.

The most important of all hedgings are the field boundaries that once made England from an aerial view look like a patchwork quilt of enclosed farmlands. These enclosures marked areas both of possession and responsibility. The living fence encompasses far more than itself. It is home and haven to wildlife, from insect and invertebrates to mammals and birds. The destruction of hedges went hand-in-hand with mass-produced crops, causing annihilation of habitat for dwellings of creatures other than mankind. This represents a serious flaw in "progress", which finally robs humans of beauty, species and birdsong. Many lyrical birds' melodies are now unknown to a whole generation, but via the hedge the healing gardener has an unsurpassable opportunity to provide a protective barrier for his property, and help to recompose nature's harmonies.

Throughout history we encounter many images of the hedge represented as a labyrinth or maze: the Cretan Minotaur's design found on coins from 1500 BC; the maze-like motifs found on Roman mosaic floors; and Native American, Indian and African carvings resembling labyrinths. The labyrinthine hedge is exemplified in the familiar maze of Hampton Court Palace's grounds laid out in 1690 for the entertainment of courtiers.

GUELDER ROSE

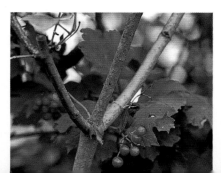

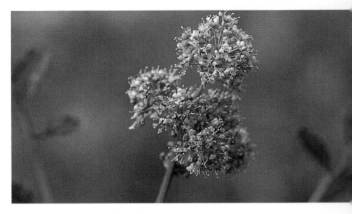

CEANOTHUS REPENS

GROWING HEDGES

The phenomenal 100-feet-high wall of beech trees at Meikleour, Scotland, forms the tallest trimmed hedge in Britain. Only grand estates can support the traditional stilt hedge – a clipped hedge with bare trunks at its base. However, shrubs and even small trees do not have to be confined to their place, especially in a small garden. A hedge need not be limited to the quick-growing privet, whitethorn, laurel, myrobella plum, or the euonymous, planted in autumn in the country and in urban areas in spring; nor the more ponderous growth of handsome box, yew or holly. A hedge, like life, is very much what you make of it. It can be greatly enhanced by the intertwining of floral climbers, such as clematis, and the pretty sight and appealing fragrance of Japanese herbal honeysuckle (*Lonicera japonica*).

In modern times of crime, burglary in particular, it is wise to grow an easily maintained and controlled, dense prickly hedge to dissuade the lawbreaker. Back garden hedges of thorny hawthorn (*Crataegus laevigata* syn. *C. oxyancantha*) and blackthorn (*Prunus spinosa*) can be cultivated. These can be interlaced with dense-growing prickly, old-fashioned shrub roses such as the hippy quartered-flowering *Rosa* 'Lanei' or sweet briar (*R. eglanteria* syn. *R. rubiginosa*), mixed with dog rose (*R. canina*). The end result should be a formidable but attractive barrier that is discouraging, yet herbally providential.

Hedges of all types and sizes may be grown not only to provide fencing, or garden divisions, but also to medicinal advantage. They give us the added bonus of exquisite colour and scent. Lavender of many differing varieties (besides *L. angustifolia*) is a plant that walks happily down the garden path with virginal blue and fragrantly scented rosemary (*Rosmarinus officinalis*).

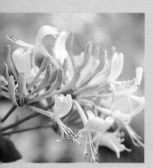

HONEYSUCKLE

"Shrubs there are,
That at the call of spring
Burst forth in blossom'd fragrance; lilacs robed
In snow-white innocence of purple pride."
Spring **from** *Seasons* **by James Thomson**
(1700-48)

MEDICINE, COLOUR AND SCENT
Californian lilac (*Ceanothus spp.*) confers a misty
vista of powdery pale blue or deep cerulean,
providing famous New Jersey tea. Its roots are versatile in respiratory afflictions, and also stimulate
the lymphatic system. Guelder rose (*Viburnum
opulus*), the astringent cramp bark used by North
American settlers, is good for cramps and body
pains. Viburnums were also employed by other
native tribes of North America for swollen glands
and mumps. They have pretty white sterile flowers,
and clusters of glossy scarlet fruits.

The cultivar, *V. opulus* 'Aureum', sheds a golden
light; the pompom variety, *V. opulus* 'Roseum', or
"snowball bush", has creamy white ball-shaped
flower heads; and *V. opulus* 'Xanthocarpum', has
translucent golden yellow berries, all growing to
around 12 feet. The black haw or stagbush
(*Viburnum prunifolium*), native to southern North
America, has blue-black berries and grows a little
taller. It is also a Native American anti-spasmodic

plant used for uterine problems and menstrual pain.

We should not overlook the powerful antiseptic and astringent properties present in myrtle's fragrant flowers (*Myrtus communis*), nor the waxed beauty of Chinese camellia (*Camellia sinensis*), which contribute a tea full of antioxidants, giving protection against heart disease, strokes and cancer. And, of course, the roses – *Rosa canina, R. eglanteria,* Cherokee R. *laevigata,* Japanese R. *rugosa* – with their multifarious healing virtues.

Why did the English herbalist John Gerard bother to say of the lilac (*Syringa vulgaris*), a plant that has seemingly little medicinal merit, "I have them growing in my garden in great plenty"? Because of its colour, and the power of the lilac's sweet, resonant perfume. It is, as the German poet Göethe said, "a flower of the heart". Its spiritual colourings, and fresh fragrance inhaled, uplift the spirits and comfort the dejected. Lilac has a never-to-be-forgotten, piercing, poignant perfume. Its purple spires are iridescent, and the flowers' ability to fade into roseate hues caused the 18th-century English poet Cowper to term them "sanguine".

An American vermifuge, tonic, anti-periodic and febrifuge, and a substitute for aloes in treatment of malaria, the aromatic lilac helps the dispirited or those waning from winter's severity. One can take every opportunity to inhale lilac's fresh fragrance on the bough; sit on a chair near it when the sun has warmed it, and revel in its healing aroma.

SYRINGA VULGARIS 'SENSATION'

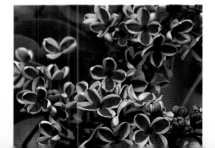

Blackthorn

Blackthorn is the burning bush of white light that disperses winter's gloom, signalling the impending spring.
The musky erotic scent of its blossoms speak to bees
and man alike of rising sap and forthcoming delights.
Believed to bloom at midnight on Christmas Eve, this
ancestor of our domestic plum provided wood for fires
and ashes scattered to fertilize the earth.

Healing and Home Uses: Psychologically, blackthorn's visual effect is ignored more than any
other of the floral realm. White is the highest
spiritual healing colour. The sight of blackthorn's
blossom and its aroma re-awakens the emotional
and mental aspects flowing from mind to body,
regenerating the physical urge for creativity.
Notoriously astringent, "Irish tea", a leaf infusion,
may be too rigorously purgative for some to
cleanse the stomach and purge the bowel, but a
weak infusion (see p.122) of blossoms [1 tsp (5
ml) flowers to 1 cup water, infused for 3-5 mins]
can assist the "spring cleaning" decongestion.
The autumnal ripe fruits, known as sloes, are
used to make strong alcoholic drinks, which
boost the circulation, raising blood pressure, and
conveying amazing warmth to the intestines.

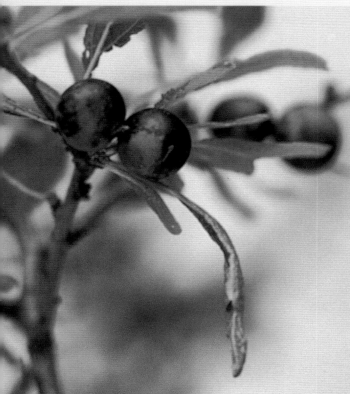

Gypsy Sloe Liqueur

4 oz (114 g) fresh-picked sloes
17 fl oz (483 ml) gin
6 fl oz (170 ml) red grape juice
1 tbsp (15 ml) lemon juice
4 heaped tbsp (60 ml) honey
¼ tsp (1¼ ml) ground clove and ½ tsp (2½ ml) nutmeg. Pick, de-stalk, rinse sloes. Warm grape juice in
pan, stir in honey, nutmeg and lemon juice. When
dissolved, cover, leave to cool. Prick sloes with fork,
place in large glass container with clove, cover with
gin. Add honey mixture, cover. Leave in warm place
for 10 days. Strain into jug, squeezing all liquid
from sloes. Discard solids, pour liquid into wine
bottle, seal. Store in cool place for 9 weeks. Decant
separate from sediment, seal. Store for 3 months.

✳ ❀ See p.133.

BLACKTHORN (PRUNUS SPINOSA)

Hawthorn

Hawthorn is a shrub or small tree highly suitable for adorning the garden. Commonly associated with Christ's crown of thorns, it symbolises hope. The Ancient Greeks carried torches of its wood to light the way for newly-weds to the bridal chamber. In Turkey a gift of a hawthorn branch implies a kiss is expected.

HAWTHORN (CRATAEGUS MONOGYNA)

Healthy Heart Tonic

Gather ½ lb (250 g) hawthorn berries. Wash thoroughly and squeeze out pips. Soak berries in 2 pt (1 lt) water overnight (covered). Pour mixture (fruits and water) into pan. Bring to boil and simmer for 10 minutes. Cool and strain into jug.

Preparation Tip: Use good plump very ripe berries, that make the pips easier to expel between thumb and first finger.

  See p.133.

Healing Uses: Always considered a "heart herb", medicinally hawthorn is an international contender of great interest to modern research. Relatively non-toxic, unlike many other plants that act upon the heart, it has a unique balancing action on the circulatory system. The berries are good antioxidants and form a cardiotonic, which both relaxes and dilates the arteries of the heart, promoting good blood-flow useful to angina. Hawthorn is a good preventive medicine, excellent for ageing hearts. It will assist insomnia of nervous origin and is good for the liver, gall bladder and digestive system.

Home Uses: In a traditional bread-and-butter sandwich, young and fresh hawthorn leaves are a good spring-clean tonic for the blood.

Shrub Roses & Hips

The pale pink "briar" dog rose (*R. canina*) grows wild in hedgerows, has a delicate perfume in summer, and with its cardinal fruits offers strength to the body in autumn. The hips of shrub roses and old-fashioned prickly roses are an offering of jewels of crimson, scarlet and vermilion to sustain our health against the dark cold days of winter.

Healing Uses: Rosehip seed oil (*R. eglanteria*) provides effective skin treatment, boosting tissue regeneration and rejuvenation. It is excellent for scars, burns and wrinkles. As a seasonal balancer for the system, scarlet dog-rose hips contain eight times as much vitamin C, weight for weight, as oranges. Diluted in water, it is still a nutritive thirst-quenching summer drink for babies and infants; a gentle remedy for diarrhoea, gastric inflammation and skin problems caused by vitamin C deficiency, and is mildly diuretic.

Home Uses: Vitamin C-rich rosehip tea made from crushed fresh or dried hip shells helps ward off colds and infections. Rosehip syrup is a versatile additive to healthfully sweeten and flavour foods, make preserves, vinegars and wine, to flavour ice-cream and add to soothing cough mixtures.

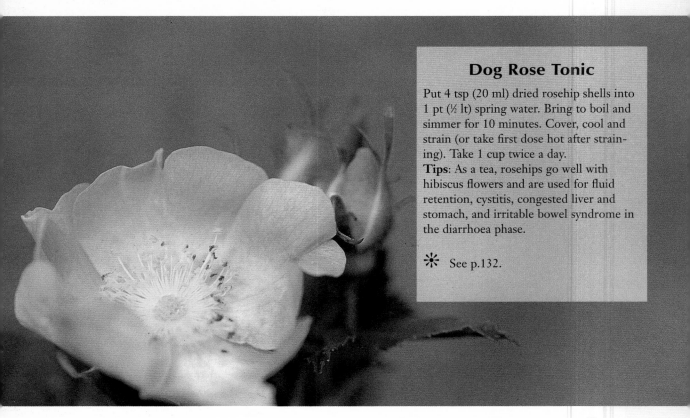

Dog Rose Tonic

Put 4 tsp (20 ml) dried rosehip shells into 1 pt (½ lt) spring water. Bring to boil and simmer for 10 minutes. Cover, cool and strain (or take first dose hot after straining). Take 1 cup twice a day.

Tips: As a tea, rosehips go well with hibiscus flowers and are used for fluid retention, cystitis, congested liver and stomach, and irritable bowel syndrome in the diarrhoea phase.

✳ See p.132.

DOG ROSE (ROSA CANINA)

40

Rosemary

With flowerets like sprinkled early morning bluey-dew in the distance, rosemary is a herb for body, mind and spirit and symbolic of fidelity and remembrance. Greek scholars wore garlands for examinations to aid their concentration and memory. In sixteenth-century England it was strewn in the law courts against "gaol fever", and was the disinfectant of French hospitals until 1930.

ROSEMARY (*ROSMARINUS OFFICINALIS*)

Gardener's Barrier Ointment for Scratches

Gently melt 4 tbsp (60 ml) vaseline in bain-marie to liquify. Add double handful of tender rosemary flower shoots. Leave to steep in hot place for 45 minutes, reheating maceration each time it solidifies. Warm to liquify and strain into sterile glass jar. When cool, before it solidifies, add 6 drops rosemary essential oil. Cool, seal, date and label. A quicker alternative is to liquify plain petroleum jelly and add maximum of 30 drops (2½ %) of rosemary essential oil to 4 tbsp (60 ml) of the jelly, just before setting.

  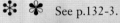 See p.132-3.

Healing Uses: Inhalations and compresses (see p.123) of the essential oil focus mental powers , relieve fatigue, nervous exhaustion, headaches and stress-related disorders. Herbal infusions (see p.122) and oil (only to be used externally) assist hypotension, muscular pain, and poor circulatory problems of arteriosclerosis. Aromatic and restorative, the herb and oil aid hepatic disorders and digestion, especially of fats. The oil in massage shifts depression.

Home Uses: Use a bath bag of rosemary to aid muscular aches and fatigue. For the complexion, add a few sprigs (or 1-3 drops of oil) to water for a steam-facial. Combine in a "tea" with lemon verbena for low spirits, or with lavender infused in the ratio of 2 parts rosemary to 1 part lavender.

Myrtle

Myrtle is a biblical plant renowned for its violet-like scent and oriental fragrant water *eau d'ange*. It is found in the Mediterranean, South-west Europe and North Africa, and throughout warmer and tropical climates worldwide. Even in Roman times myrtle was the emblem of love. An Arabian tale narrates that Adam offered a sprig of myrtle when declaring love to Eve.

Healing Uses: The oil is used for bronchitis and generally for respiratory complaints. The leaves, fruits and oil of the herb are an astringent, and antiseptic tonic. The herb is used internally for dry coughs, bronchial congestion, sinusitis, urinary infections and vaginal discharge. Externally, the oil helps periodontal infections, acne, oily skin, asthma, bronchitis, catarrhal conditions and chronic coughs and haemorrhoids.

Home Uses: The oil is mild enough to be administered externally to children in massage for coughs and chest ailments. As preventive medicine a dried powdered buds infusion]½ tsp (2½ ml) to 1 cup of water] helps urinary infections. It can be added to meats as a spice, especially where infections are recurrent. Pulverized leaves and flowers added to ointment (see p.125) are good for skin blemishes.

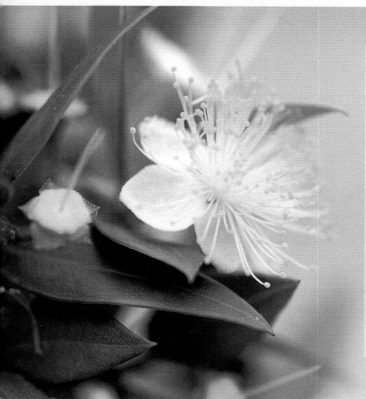

Myrtle Cleansing Mask

1 tsp (5 ml) beeswax
1 tbsp (15 ml) lanolin or sweet almond oil
2 fl oz (50 ml) orange flower or rose water
1 tbsp (15 ml) fuller's earth or powdered oatmeal
1 tsp (5 ml) powdered myrtle dried flowers and leaves
9 drops *M. communis* essential oil
In bain-marie, melt beeswax and lanolin or almond oil over gentle heat, stirring continuously. Remove from stove; add orange or rose water until mixture has cooled. Add fuller's earth/oatmeal, mixing to smooth paste. Immediately before application to face, add myrtle oil. Cleanse face; cover eyes with cucumber or cotton-wool eye-pads soaked in herbal infusion or cold water for 20-30 minutes. Remove with warm water, cold-splash face with water or elderflower infusion.

MYRTLE (MYRTUS COMMUNIS)

Lavender

The Garden Healer will appreciate lavender's dry cultivation habit, whether as a small hedging or divider of space. In droughty conditions, its love of hot dry areas makes it a candidate for a gravel garden, where it can be grown together with like-minded ornamental alliums, cistus, thymes and other remedial herbs.

LAVENDER (LAVANDULA ANGUSTIFOLIA)

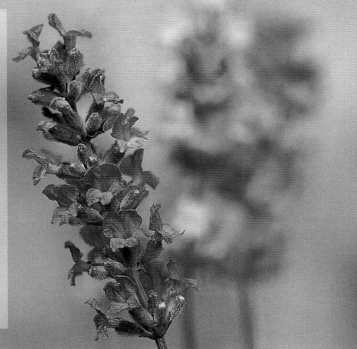

Menopause

Lavender essential oil happens to be one of nature's providences that can help menopausal symptoms. In particular its rejuvenative attributes are tailor-made to assist the menopause. The cessation of menstruation can occur at any age, usually between the mid-thirties and mid-fifties. A change occurs in the balance of sex hormones sometimes leading to "hot flushes", palpitations and dryness of the vaginal mucous membranes. Emotional disturbances, depression and sleeplessness from night sweats can be alleviated by taking oestrogenic hormones in HRT (hormone replacement therapy).
For those women unsuited to HRT lavender oil can assist with balancing of the emotions.

Healing and Home Uses: Lavender has a very wide variety of uses, largely through its "balancing" oil. The power of its colour and scent should never be underestimated. The essential oil in massage is good for lumbago, sprains, rheumatism and muscular aches and pains. Massage and/or vaporize the oil to assist nervous-related asthma and bronchitis. It is a circulatory stimulant with analgesic and strong anti-depressant effects – useful for insomnia, irritability, headaches and some migraines. Lavender tea aids cramps, colic, dyspepsia, flatulence and, for some, nausea: 1 tsp (5 ml) to 1 cup of water. A wash will help cystitis. The feminine aspect of the oil is used in dysmenorrhoea, leucorrhea, hypertension, nervous tension, PMS, and stress-related conditions.

Camellia

Named after George Joseph Kamel, a Jesuit pharma-cist, camellia was introduced to Europe from China in 1639 AD, where the tea, *Camellia sinensis,* or black tea, has been drunk for over 3,000 years. Most temperate gardens can find a hot spot for "the roses of Japan", either in the ground or in a tub against a warm wall.

Healing and Home Uses: *Camellia sinensis* should be made from the shoot tips. Ayurvedic medicine employs *C. sinensis* as an astringent, a stimulant nerve and cardiac tonic, for the diges-tion and fatigue, as well as externally to relieve insect bites and inflammations. Research has proved it inhibits tumour formation and growth, which may protect against some cancers. The aromatic buds and leaves contain flavonoids and vitamin C and are bactericidal, useful in stomach infections such as dysentery and gastroenteritis, and are used in moderation for short periods only. Conversely, excess dosage causes nervous and dyspeptic symptoms, such as giddiness, pal-pitations, constipation and insomnia. An infusion (see p.122) is a good febrifuge to counter effects from too much sun. Apply as a wash for sunburn and cold compress for headaches.

Camellia Compress

Pick 2 tbsp (30 ml) of camellia shoots and place in pyrex jug. Pour over 1 pt (½ lt) boiling water. Cover and allow to stand until cooled. Use cotton-wool swabs to dab on areas of body affected by sunburn. Dip a wide strip of lint into liquid and apply to temples. Repeat a few times whenever lint becomes heated or dries out. For a recumbent person, soak strip of sterile cotton wool in liquid, place between muslin, place over forehead and gently bind around head with strip of clean bandage.

TEA (CAMELLIA SINENSIS)

Common Broom

The Greeks gave broom its generic name *kytisos*, which describes the habitat of this ornamental shrub. Common broom *(Cytisus scoparius)* grows wild on native heaths, in woodlands and on waste grounds of Europe, and flourishes in the warmer climes of North Africa and Western Asia. Its blossom, which appears in May and June, is golden and vanilla-fragranced.

BROOM (CYTISUS SCOPARIUS)

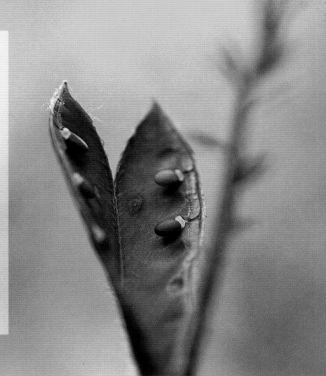

Broom-Scented Soap

Collect and cleanse 2 tbsp (30 ml) broom flowers (not set for seed). Put in heat-proof glass container and add 2 fl oz (50 ml) hot sweet almond oil; leave to infuse and cool. Press down and weight clean lid that fits inside container to help extract aroma. Take bar of pure soap (shave or break up) and place in bain-marie to dissolve. When the soap has liquified, remove from heat, allow to cool, but not set, before adding macerated floral oil. If you do not possess moulds, use both sides of old travel soap box. Pour in perfumed liquid and allow to set.

✳ ✱ ✿   see pp.132-3.

Healing Uses: A bitter narcotic herb, the sight and scent of glorious golden broom is very healing. Walking through it, or sitting beside its fragrance, can waft away headaches.

Home Uses: Apart from common broom, there is the pineapple aroma of Moroccan broom (*C. battandieri*). The Tenerife broom, *C supranubius* syn. *C. fragrans*, is a less hardy cousin, covered in emerald-green foliage all year with scented pinkish-white blossoms. A decoction (see p.123) of the flowers (*C. scoparius* only) added to soap, is reminiscent of recipes for scented ox fat favoured by Ancient Egyptians, who wore such cones on their heads, allowing them to dissolve and drip down to perfume their bodies at banquets.

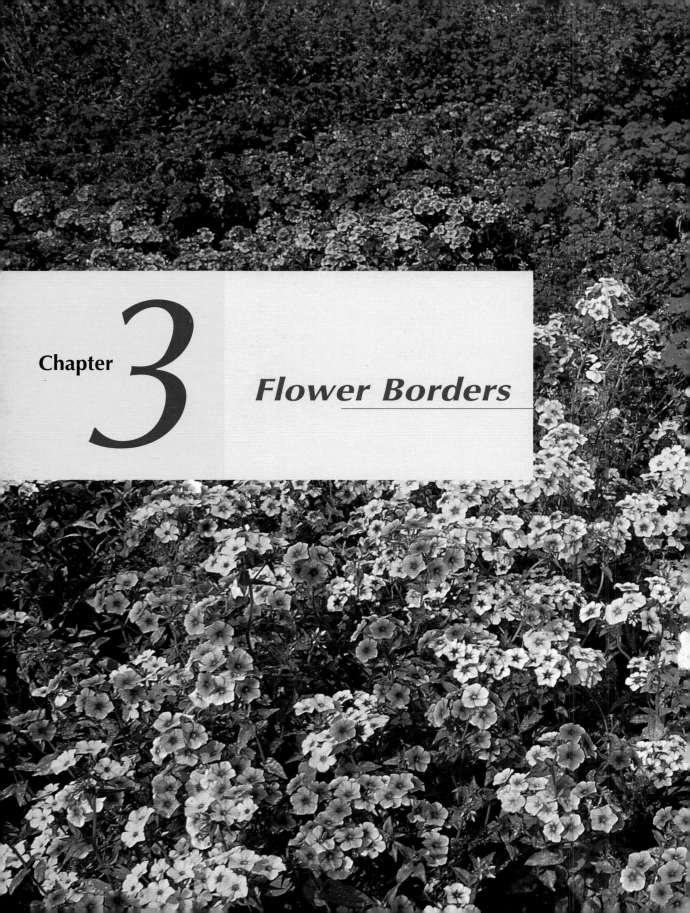

Chapter

3

Flower Borders

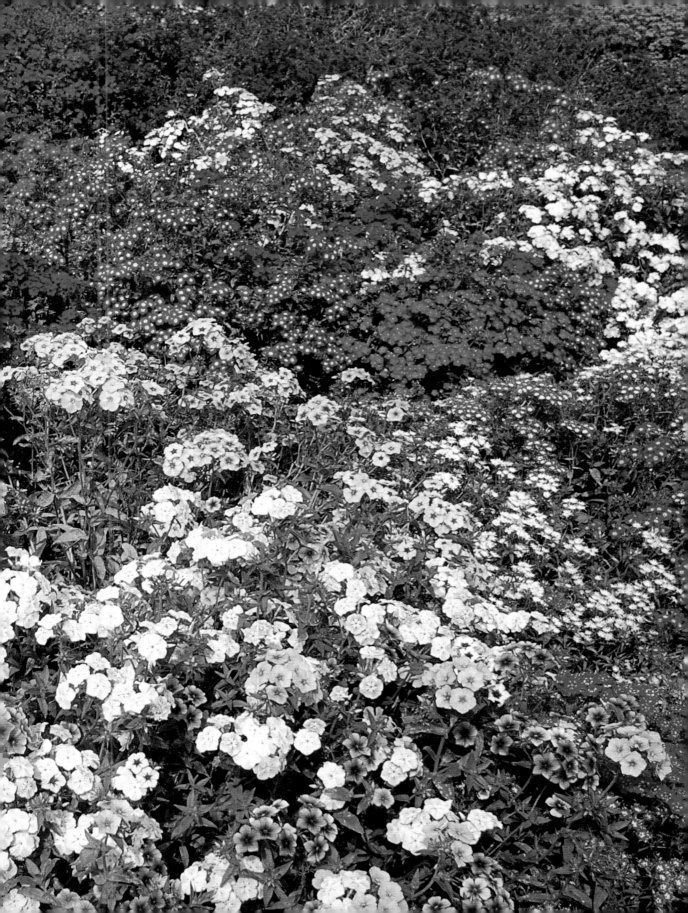

Flower borders

We need not wonder at the universality of some species, why many different plants are common to the same generic family, because originally the earth's landmass was all one. The movement of the tectonic plates continues in motion, especially of "the rooftop of the world" in North India and Nepal. The ability of plant organisms to adapt and genetically alter has accommodated the establishment of different species of the same genus worldwide.

New species secreted in cut-off micro-climates of the world can add to the interest of the flower border. For instance, the recent importation of flowering plants from South Africa, such as geraniums (*Pelargoniums*), can enhance the European gardeners' choice of plants to combat the effects of global warming. These flowers are likely not only to gladden the eye, but help us fight the ills of a future generation.

Whilst trees may represent the masculine principle in the garden, flowers might be seen as the feminine "pretty maids all in a row". There is much to excite the mind and imagination in the flower border: from colourful friendly pansy masks and fresh-faced violets (*Violas*) to aesthetic architectural plants, like artichoke (with its metallic, blue-purple leaves) and sunbursts of sunflowers (*Helianthus annuus*); from multi-coloured hollyhocks (*Alcea rosea*), to sun-spangled iridescent aromatic irises (*Iris pallida* and *I. germanica* 'Florentina'). *Delphinium staphisagria* and *D. brunonianum* can provide an insecticide once used to eradicate lice. Another fine flower is indigo aconite, powerfully musk-scented, erotic and poisonous, and still widely used in medicine and homoeopathy.

Many familiar flowers have hidden talents, such as climbers like the Australian clematis

CHEDDAR PINK

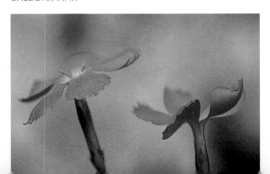

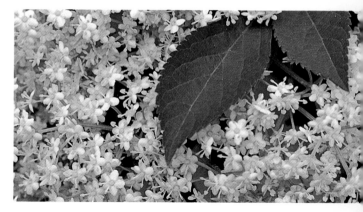

ELDERFLOWERS

species (*Clematis glycinoides*), an Aboriginal traditional remedy for colds and headaches; or passionflowers (*Passiflora incarnata*), a tonic of the Houma tribe of North America. There are also the familiar dahlias (*D.* x *hortensis*), yielding laevulose, extracted in Germany for diabetic sugar. Others to inspire are wallflowers (*Erysimum cheiri*) with their heart-warming aroma; Sweet William (*Dianthus barbatus*), a native of Southern Germany, acclaimed by Emperor Charles V's physician for its clovine healing scent; and the much-loved carnation (*D. caryophyllus*). Finally, the fringed pink (*D. superbus*), used in China and Japan, and a reliever of kidney complaints; mysterious flamboyant paeonies (*Paeonia lactiflora* and *P. officinalis*); and the kaleidoscopic panoply of poppies.

Fragrance alone can help sustain psychological balance in today's busy life. Flowers offer a wonderful world of pungent odours and scented sights – a perception perhaps more

readily appreciated by the blind. Babies can greatly benefit from being in the environs of the smell of lavender and roses. The scent of honeysuckle and violets, in particular, may stir the psyche of the sensitive. The romance of the night is captured by night-scented stocks (*Matthiola langipetala* subsp. *bicornis*), royal jasmine (*Jasminum grandiflorum*), and tobacco plants (*Nicotiana spp.*) – all with rich, clinging, provocative and highly intoxicating perfumes.

Some flowers are aphrodisiacs, like the pink-flowered morning glory (*Ipomoea mauritiana*), an Ayurvedic sexual stimulant and rejuvenative tonic, and the animal-musk-scented elderflowers, often found lurking near the compost heap. There are also roses, freesias and the piercingly fragrant lily-of-the-valley.

The flower border is the point at which small flowering trees, shrubs, tall plants, vegetables and herbs can companionably meet and fraternize. It is essentially the junction at

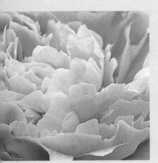

DOUBLE PINK PEONY

" *O Flowers, they are all the
time travelling like comets, and
they come into our ken for a day,
… and slowly vanish again. And
we, we must take them on the
wing, and let them go. … Flowers
are just a swift motion, a coloured
gesture; that is their loveliness. And
that is love.*"
**Poem *Fidelity* from *Pansies*
collection, 1929, D.H. Lawrence
(1885-1930)**

which gather the senses of sight, smell and touch.
A strategic self-cycling water feature will enhance
this symphony of the senses with sound, creating a
haven for the care-worn. Raised flower beds will
allow the partially sighted, as well as those physically impaired, to enjoy the delights of gardening.

The Garden Healer has the widest artistic palate
from which to create a personal, practical and
remedial picture. Back-drops of Philadelphus and
Daphne, and many other aromatic shrubs extend
that perspective. Sweet geraniums (*Pelargonium
spp.*) can titillate taste-buds with their different aromas of: oranges, 'Charity' and 'Prince of Orange';
citrus, 'Lemon Fancy'; rose, 'Attar of Roses' and
'Lady Plymouth'; and also the scents of cedar,
cinnamon and nutmeg.

We can sculpt creeping thymes and chamomile
into cushions for wall-seats, or fill a cement
Roman-style chaise-longue for curative reclination.
Chives and pinks are excellent herbal edgings to sit
at the feet of roses. All alliums are happy to cohabit
with them, and red-purpled chard will colourfully
fill a drift. Given encouragement, vibrant lemon,

orange and scarlet nasturtiums will grow beside even the darkest yew hedge, lending medicinal and culinary companionship where no other flower desires to be cultivated.

Unless wishing it so, the Garden Healer need not be slave to fashion's dictates, weaving a tapestry swatched in hostas and variegated foliage alone. Be bold like "the lilies of the field", found painted on walls of Cretan palaces (*c.*1500 BC). An emblem of Greek Herculean purity, lilies stamp their mark and set their royal feet in woodland and estate alike, sporting every colour drifting on a musical scale of perfume.

The lily family offers a splendid array of flowers. There are the sweetly scented Canadian meadow lily (*Lilium canadense*); the golden-rayed lily (*L. auratum*), wild from Japan, with its penetrating spicy perfume and *L. iridollae* from Alabama with a soft sweet fragrance. Others are the regal lily *(L. regale)* with a Tibetan honeysuckle redolence; the nightly fragrant Martagon lily (*L. martagon*) of Southern Europe; and the Easter lily (*L. longiflorum*) of delicate jasmine aroma.

The colours, scents and textures of plants are subtle and infinite. Follow your heart and remedial intentions and it is almost certain that you will produce a classic flower border belonging in any sized garden which is never out of vogue. The palate is the whole myriad spectrum at your artistic service, and the garden, your own canvas, which you can individually create to take on a wonderful curative and spiritually satisfying adventure.

HEARTSEASE PANSIES

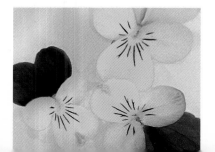

Honeysuckle

Regaled by English poets, honeysuckle's sweet nectar exemplifies the blessings of the Chinese New Year – robust health, love and happiness. Longevity is the blessing of its "tea", popular in China and Japan. It is identified as the third flower of the Song of Solomon, the lily among thorns, and in ancient folklore it protects against evil spirits.

Healing Uses: Its scent is warming and healing to the emotions. Its meditative flowers are the visualization colour of holy creativity. The cooling flowers are added to lotions for skin inflammations, infections, rashes and sores. Internally, it is used for rheumatoid arthritis and childhood infections such as chicken pox and measles.

Home Uses: Honeysuckle makes a rustic floral wine fit for the gods. It is a herb "tea" much used by the elderly in the Orient. Add ½ tsp (2½ ml) of fresh honeysuckle flowers to 1 cup of green tea to stimulate the circulation and the flow of oxygen to the brain.

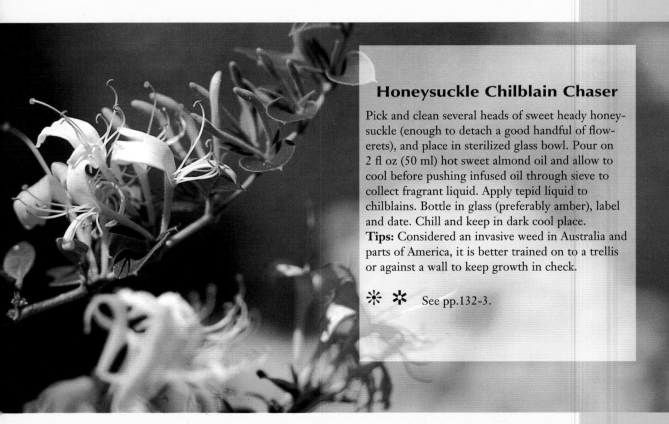

Honeysuckle Chilblain Chaser

Pick and clean several heads of sweet heady honeysuckle (enough to detach a good handful of flowerets), and place in sterilized glass bowl. Pour on 2 fl oz (50 ml) hot sweet almond oil and allow to cool before pushing infused oil through sieve to collect fragrant liquid. Apply tepid liquid to chilblains. Bottle in glass (preferably amber), label and date. Chill and keep in dark cool place.
Tips: Considered an invasive weed in Australia and parts of America, it is better trained on to a trellis or against a wall to keep growth in check.

✳ ✳ See pp.132-3.

JAPANESE HONEYSUCKLE (LONICERA JAPONICA)

Catmint/Catnip

Catmint takes its common name from its attraction for and stimulatory effect upon cats. Roman *Nepeta* has decorative, culinary and medicinal uses. It is a pretty powder blue or white flowering border edging plant, traditionally set in front of lavender and roses. It encourages bees and discourages vermin, and planted near vegetables deters flea beetles. The leaf and flowering tops contain vitamin C.

CATMINT (NEPETA X FAASENII)

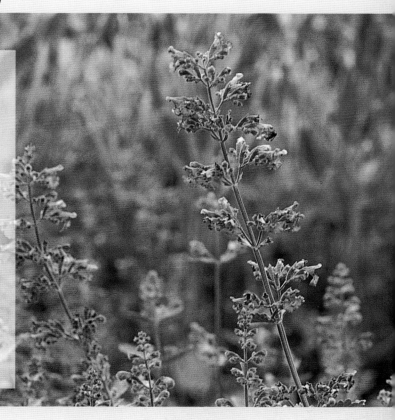

Children's Colds & Flu Remedy

Gentle catnip (*Nepeta cataria*) is suitable for children's colds, flu, indigestion and colic. It induces sleep and perspiration, but does not increase body temperature, and is mildly sedative.

1 tbsp (15 ml) fresh catmint leaves
1 pt (½ lt) boiling water
Put leaves into pot, pour over boiling liquid and cover. Stand for 10 minutes and strain before use. Drink warm.
Preparation Tips: Wash fresh material expelling all dirt and insects. Tear the leaves for maximum effect. For children mix catnip with elderflower and sweeten with honey.

Healing Uses: Before tea reached Britain from China, catmint's leaves were used as "tea" and drunk with milk and sugar. K'Eogh's *An Irish Herbal* (1735) recommended it to facilitate urination and menstruation, opening blockages of the lungs and womb; also, as an aid to internal bruises and shortness of breath. Chinese medicine uses catnip (*N. cataria*) for haemorrhages, post-natal bleeding, heavy menstruation, colds, measles and nettle rash. A professional tincture may be made into an ointment for haemorrhoids or into an alcoholic "rub" for rheumatism and arthritis.
Home Uses: An infusion (see p.122) relieves cold and fever symptoms, settles the stomach and alleviates headaches that accompany gastric upsets. It is soporific, sudorific, and an aid to digestive infections.

Forget-me-not

The heavenly face of the forget-me-not has lent its celestial colour to "blue", although it appears in pink, melting into shades of lavender. It is a self-seeding plant scattered in gardens worldwide. The forget-me-not family provides us with the cerulean blue-flowered borage and comfrey, the Roman's uniting "knitbone", both once used as pot herbs and in medicine.

Healing Uses: From its valiant persistent growth in the garden it is easy to see why forget-me-not shares with borage a strong affinity for the respiratory organs, and on a psychological note compares in floral essence with John Gerard's "I Borage, bring always courage". Possessing demulcent, emollient and cooling qualities, it can be used externally as an infusion (see p.122) for cooling skin.

Home Uses: For chest pain accompanying pleurisy, a forget-me-not poultice can be a helpful means of pain reduction and pleural decongestion. Pleurisy is a serious condition, sometimes recurrent, always associated with some other disease in the lung, chest wall, diaphragm or abdomen. Caused by inflammation of the pleura, usually due to pneumonia in the underlying lung, there is pain on deep breathing.

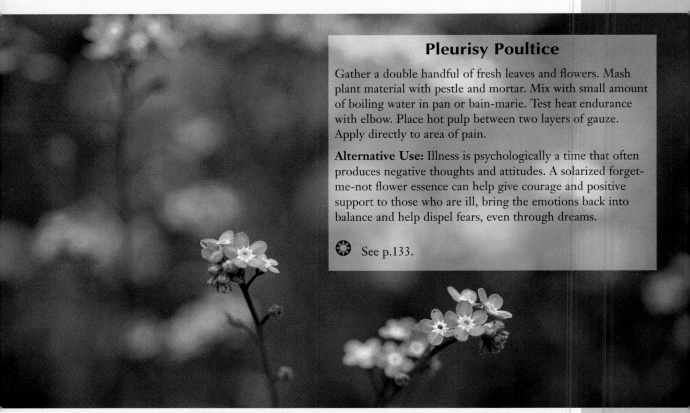

Pleurisy Poultice

Gather a double handful of fresh leaves and flowers. Mash plant material with pestle and mortar. Mix with small amount of boiling water in pan or bain-marie. Test heat endurance with elbow. Place hot pulp between two layers of gauze. Apply directly to area of pain.

Alternative Use: Illness is psychologically a time that often produces negative thoughts and attitudes. A solarized forget-me-not flower essence can help give courage and positive support to those who are ill, bring the emotions back into balance and help dispel fears, even through dreams.

✵ See p.133.

FOREGET-ME-NOT (MYOSOTIS SYLVATICA)

Mallow/Hollyhock

The bee-loud hollyhock, or high mallow, ranges from the maroon-black 'Nigra' garden varieties to colourful nineteenth-century showy splendours of double-floral delights. Cousin to the mallow, it remains in our gardens as one of childhood's towering wonders of the plant world and is, like marigold, child's play to propagate.

BLACK ALTHAEA OFFICINALIS 'NIGRA'

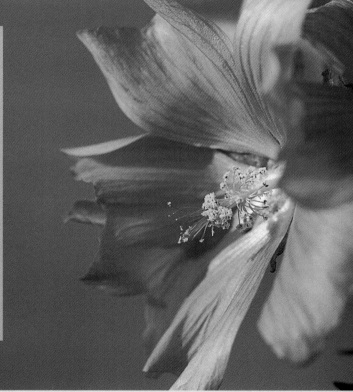

Gastric Ulcer Soothing Syrup

Large double handful fresh marshmallow leaves (*Althaea officinalis*)
2 pt (1 lt) spring water
Pick and clean leaves, place in pan, with enough water to cover, and simmer for 20-30 minutes. Strain and push through jelly bag when cool.
To each measured pint of liquid add 12 oz (350 g) sugar. Returning liquid and sugar to pan, simmer for 10-15 minutes. Bottle, label and date or freeze.

Preparation Tips: The root mucilage, which contains asparagin and has diuretic properties, is strongest in winter. Use gentle *Alcea rosea* for children's gastric upsets as it is milder.

 See p.133.

Healing uses: Emollient and demulcent, hollyhock makes a good mouthwash for early onset of gingivitis. The Bedouin use decoctions internally for the digestion and externally to soothe inflamed skin. Medicinally the roots are employed internally for gastritis, inflammation and ulceration of the digestive tract, and as a cough expectorant; the leaves are used for urinary infections and respiratory complaints.

Externally, poultices are used for boils, abscesses, insect bites, splinters and other minor injuries, and on occasion mastitis.
Home Uses: Use mallow cream for dry eczema; a root poultice (see p.125) for minor wounds; leaf compress (see p.123) for burns; and a root syrup for an irritating cough and sore throat. Toss young leaves and flowers into salads, or steam young leaves for gastric problems.

Poppy

Rich in folklore, the poppy is universally loved by all nations. The family roots of opium poppies (*Papaver somniferum*) lie with the archaic Sumerians and Chaldeans. The warriors of Egyptian Thebes employed the field poppy (*Papaver rhoeas*) medicinally and the Assyrians christened her "Daughter of the Field". The precious jewel of the Himalayan poppy (*Meconopsis*) is a sapphire transported from the rooftop of the world and planted into the hub of modern life.

Ayurvedic Poppy Drink

A good cure for diarrhoea:
Crush 1-2 tsp (5-10 ml) ripe dried poppy seeds (*P. rhoeas*). Place them in pan with 1 cupful of spring water. Boil mixture, add a pinch of carminative nutmeg. Blend and then drink.

Incontinence

Incontinence is the inappropriate or involuntary passage of urine, most commonly bed-wetting. Stress incontinence results from the leaking of urine when coughing or straining. It is often found in women with weakened pelvic muscles after childbirth. Overflow incontinence most commonly occurs in old men from an obstruction or neurological conditions affecting bladder control. Urge incontinence is leakage of urine accompanied by an intense desire to pass water with failure of restraint.

Incontinence Tea

1-2 tsp (5-10 ml) dried *Eschscholzia californica* herb (for adults)
½ tsp (2 ½ ml) of above (for children)
Put herb in pot and pour over 1 cup boiled water. Cover and infuse for 10 minutes.

Tip: Collect dried *P. rhoeas* seeds as they occur and keep in sealed container. Grow *Eschscholzia californica* in full sun and cut for harvesting when in full flower.

Healing Uses: Poppies' flowers speak to the Garden Healer with their gift of chromatherapy (colour healing), from base chakra sexual red energy to spiritual blue. Medicine uses *P. somniferum* products in many proprietary ways to relieve pain and suffering. Its ripe culinary seeds and oil, *huile d'oeillette*, is favoured in the Middle East, whilst Europeans use the digestive seeds of *Papaver rhoeas* and its flowers to colour medicine and wine. Non-narcotic, analgesic, antispasmodic and sedative *Eschscholzia californica*, related to *P. somniferum*, treats physical and psychological problems of children.

Home Uses: Collect ripe pungent seeds (*P. rhoeas*) and sprinkle on bread, cakes and biscuits, as a good astringent for the intestines. The seeds alleviate nervous digestive disorders, such as diarrhoea in children and adults, and abdominal pain. Pain-relieving and relaxing, the whole herb of non-narcotic *Eschscholzia californica* is sudorific and helps incontinence, particularly in children, assisting nervous tension, anxiety and insomnia. A syrup made from the petals of *P. rhoeas* can be drunk to quell pain and quieten disturbed feelings. Use of the seeds is not recommended for people with IBS, or other similar conditions.

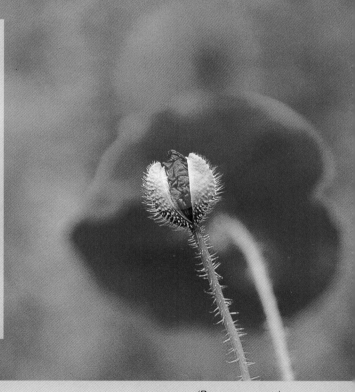

Analgesic Syrup

¼ lb (125 g) caster sugar
150 ml (15 fl oz) water
juice of half lemon
a drop of orange food colouring (optional)
double handful of *E. californica* aerial parts

Place plant material in heatproof bowl. Put sugar in pan; cover with water, lemon juice and colouring. Place over moderate heat, stirring until sugar has dissolved; bring to boil and simmer for 5 mins. Pour over plant material; cover and leave overnight. Strain and decant into sterilized bottle, seal, label and date. Dilute with spring water - 2 tsp (10 ml) to 1 wine glass (2 fl oz) to serve before bed time. For toothache 1 tsp (5 ml) undiluted is a good analgesic.

 See p.133.

FIELD POPPY (PAPAVER RHOEAS)

Alchemilla

Known as Lady's Mantle, Alchemilla is derived from the Arabic *alkemelych*, meaning "alchemy". This explains its ancient use in mystical potions and more modern reputation as a magical "mother's little helper". Before the Pill's invention, it was used to regulate periods, ease menopausal symptoms and gynaecological inflammations from the Orient to the Occident.

Healing Uses: The status of Alchemilla has waned and lost fashionability, but it is nonetheless efficacious for menstrual disorders and as an astringent tonic for the digestive system, usefully employed to check diarrhoea in gastroenteritis. Externally, it staunches wounds, clears acne and softens dry skin.

Home Uses: A double strength infusion (see p.122) taken three times daily will help to reduce period pains and excessive bleeding. Apply an infusion or stronger decoction for inflamed eyes, in a cold compress (see p.123), or to arrest bleeding and reduce swelling. The astringent leaves are useful in a facial steam or their decoction can be added to creams and lotions (see p.125), and infused for vaginal washes, vulval itching, and for a post-extraction of teeth mouthwash.

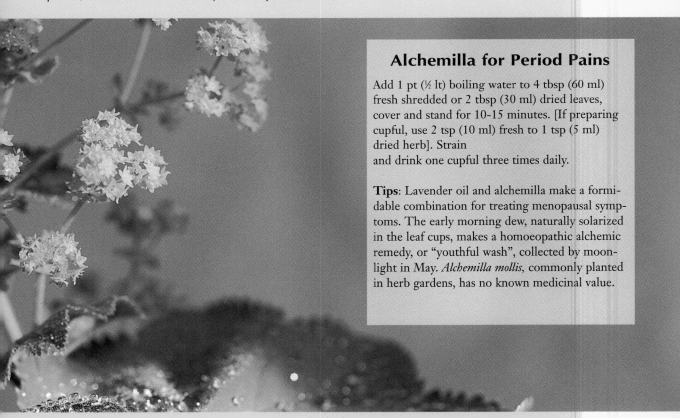

Alchemilla for Period Pains

Add 1 pt (½ lt) boiling water to 4 tbsp (60 ml) fresh shredded or 2 tbsp (30 ml) dried leaves, cover and stand for 10-15 minutes. [If preparing cupful, use 2 tsp (10 ml) fresh to 1 tsp (5 ml) dried herb]. Strain and drink one cupful three times daily.

Tips: Lavender oil and alchemilla make a formidable combination for treating menopausal symptoms. The early morning dew, naturally solarized in the leaf cups, makes a homoeopathic alchemic remedy, or "youthful wash", collected by moonlight in May. *Alchemilla mollis*, commonly planted in herb gardens, has no known medicinal value.

LADY'S MANTLE (ALCHEMILLA XANTHOCLORA)

Madonna Lily

Recorded in hieroglyphics and favoured by the Ancient Greeks and Romans for unguents and bathing, *Lilium candidum* was dedicated to the "purity" of the Madonna by the Christian Church. The source of the fabulously perfumed Oil of Lilies common to India and Persia, the Madonna lily has been cultivated in European gardens for over three centuries. In French heraldry the lily is a symbol of divinity, purity, abundance and love.

MADONNA LILY (*LILIUM CANDIDUM*)

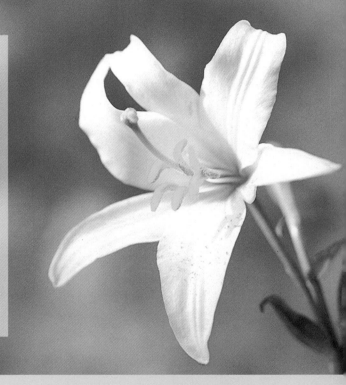

Skin-scar Prevention Lotion

3 tbsp (15 ml) fresh lily bulb
1 pt (½ lt) boiling milk

Put the lily bulb in bowl and pour over boiling liquid. Stand for 10 minutes, cool and strain before use. Label and date.

Preparation Tips: Bulbs collected in August may be used dried and fresh. To dry, strip off scales separately and spread on papered shelves in a warm room for about ten days and finish off in an oven, when it has been turned off and is cooling. Lotions are best kept in amber or blue glass bottles in a cool dark place or refrigerator, against deterioration.

Healing Uses: The heather-honey scent of lilies in mid-summer sun offers psychological comfort and is a stabilizing healer. Demulcent, astringent, and highly mucilaginous, bulbs boiled in milk or water have been used externally for ulcers and inflammation. Made into ointment, the bulbs eradicate corns and remove pain and inflammation from scalds and burns without scarring.

Home Uses: Precious to the gardener, a bulb infusion (see p.122) boiled in milk will produce a lotion for scalds and burns, and suitable for cosmetic application to the skin. Fresh blooms may be macerated (see p.124) in sweet almond oil or cider vinegar to produce a lotion for bruises, similar to arnica or calendula.

Phlox

An old-fashioned beloved of the herbaceous border, phlox have never ceased to be seen in the gardens of the great and the good. The cool, mop-headed perennials have, in some cases, scent of an acquired taste. *Phlox paniculata* has the new-mown hay and sweeter fragrance. *P. maculata* is one of the most highly scented.

Healing Uses: Ancient Greeks used *Polemonium caeruleum* with showy blue flowers for dysentery. False Jacob's Ladder, American Greek Valerian, or abscess root (*Polemonium reptans*), is a slightly bitter and acrid slender root. Used dried, it is an astringent and alternative diaphoretic and expectorant. The drug has been administered to treat feverish inflammatory cases of bronchitis and for treating laryngitis.

Home Uses: As an adult alternative remedy, the rootstock in wine can be used sparingly for febrile bronchitis where there is need to produce perspiration in inflammatory conditions. Bronchial fever is where the bronchi are inflamed and headache with a dry fever is present. By encouraging perspiration, the rootstock can alleviate fever and lower temperature.

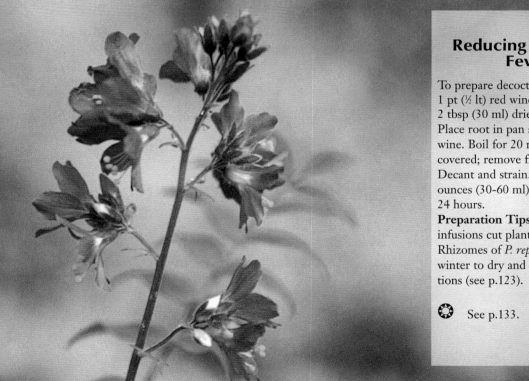

Reducing Bronchial Fevers

To prepare decoction in wine:
1 pt (½ lt) red wine
2 tbsp (30 ml) dried root
Place root in pan and cover with wine. Boil for 20 minutes. Keep covered; remove from heat to cool. Decant and strain. Take 1 to 2 fluid ounces (30-60 ml), 2-3 times over 24 hours.
Preparation Tips: For *P. caeruleum* infusions cut plants in summer. Rhizomes of *P. reptans* are lifted in winter to dry and store for decoctions (see p.123).

✵ See p.133.

JACOB'S LADDER (POLEMONIUM CAERULEUM)

Rose

The scent of a garden rose is at the heart of our very being, expressing the soft sweet petals and the thorns of life's unfolding. This queen of flowers was born of two parents, one from Persia and the other China. The rose was hallowed by Persian King Darius and Roman Emperor Nero. It was a basic ingredient of their soldiers' medicine chests, and its essence was carried in conquerors' hearts and eaten in their foods and wine.

APOTHECARY'S ROSE (ROSA GALLICA VAR. OFFICINALIS)

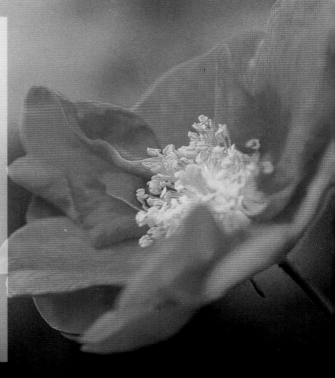

Rose Moisturizing Cream

3 tbsp (45 ml) rosewater
1 tsp (5 ml) beeswax
1 tbsp (15 ml) sweet almond oil
1 tsp (5 ml) lanolin
6 drops rose essential oil/absolute
½ tsp (2½ ml) wheat germ oil
3 tbsp (45 ml) rosewater
¼ tsp (1¼ ml) borax
In bain-marie, melt lanolin and beeswax, stirring all the while. Warm almond and wheat-germ oils gently and beat into mixture.
Dissolve borax into warmed rosewater and slowly add to mixture. Beat until cool, dropping in rose oil as mixture thickens. Store in jar, sealed, dated and labelled. Suitable for all skins.
Tip: A tiny bud of cotton-wool with 1 drop of rose oil taped into the left upper outer ear will assist insomnia. Do not use ear-bed method for insomnia on very young children.

Healing Uses: The rose, a metaphysician of perfume and flavour, celebrates the senses. Its profound scent and beauteous sight are emotionally uplifting, relieving depression, insomnia and stress. Aphrodisiac rose water's fragrance contains a euphoric which can affect attraction and orgasm, and is useful for frigidity or impotence. Cherokee rose, "jing ying zi", used in Ayurvedic medicine, is employed for the genito-urinary system and gynaecological complaints.

Home Uses: Apart from frequent inhalation of roses' perfume, bathe in rose oil mixed with a rosehip maceration (see p.124). Rich in vitamin C it is excellent for dry skin and sensitive complexions, and makes a good massage oil for difficult menstruation. Scented rose petals are edible raw for salads and can also be used in jams, vinegars and sorbets.

Sunflower

Aztecs decorated themselves with the sunflower's golden sunburst, replicating it in jewellery and patterns for over 3,000 years. In the 16th century it was brought from South America to Europe, where this remarkable "soul food" plant has been a commercial success since the 18th century. It is grown in Holland for marshland reclamation and in Germany and Siberia for oil.

Healing Uses: In Russian medicine, the seeds are used for bronchial infections, as discovered by a female Siberian healer, and the whole plant for tuberculosis and malaria (the sunflower stems and heads are macerated in vodka, to sweat). This nutritious herb lowers blood cholesterol levels and soothes irritated tissues. It is used as a carrier oil and in liniments for rheumatic complaints and muscular aches.

Home Uses: Most commonly employed as a cooking oil, the sunflower's shelled kernels, raw or roasted, are eaten worldwide and are a children's favourite. Raw buds and seed sprouts can be added to salads, or the buds steamed and served as a starter. Culinary use of the oil helps to lower blood pressure. Cosmetically, the oil is used in baths, face creams, masks and massage.

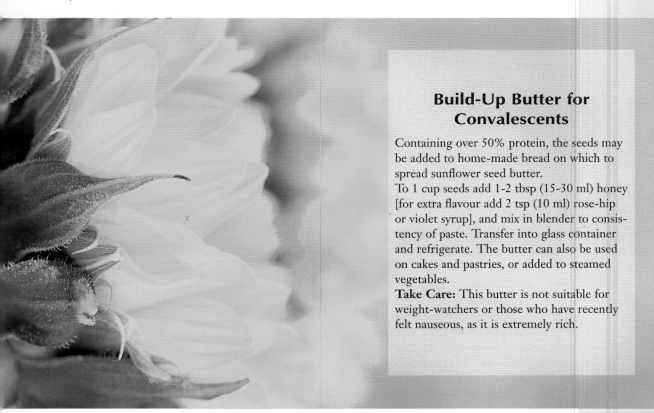

Build-Up Butter for Convalescents

Containing over 50% protein, the seeds may be added to home-made bread on which to spread sunflower seed butter.

To 1 cup seeds add 1-2 tbsp (15-30 ml) honey [for extra flavour add 2 tsp (10 ml) rose-hip or violet syrup], and mix in blender to consistency of paste. Transfer into glass container and refrigerate. The butter can also be used on cakes and pastries, or added to steamed vegetables.

Take Care: This butter is not suitable for weight-watchers or those who have recently felt nauseous, as it is extremely rich.

SUNFLOWER (HELIANTHUS ANNUUS)

Violet

The violet was first chronicled as a medicinal herb in the Ancient Egyptian *Ebers papyri* nearly 2,000 years ago. Grown the world over, the sweet violet of Mohammed has scented wines and garnished foods down the centuries. Its form was symbolic of the love between Napoleon and Josephine, his guiding star. Queen Victoria had 3,000 violet plants specially grown at Windsor to fulfil her passion for the flowers.

SWEET VIOLET (VIOLA ODORATA)

Children's Cough Syrup

Make violet flower decoction (see p.123). Take 1 pt (570 ml) violet decoction and bring slowly to boil. Stir in 2-4 tbsp (30-60 ml) honey, until mixture becomes syrupy. Cool and decant into dark glass bottle. Seal, label, date and store in refrigerator.
Take 1-2 tsp (5-10 ml) night and morning.
Tip: For adults make double-strength decoction.

✪ See p.133.

Healing Uses: Violet soothes many conditions, from hangover to headaches and influenza. The syrup, a gentle laxative, is especially useful for children and for treating respiratory disorders. Violet leaves have a European reputation for treating tumours, benign and cancerous.
Home Uses: Taken internally infusions (see p.122) help nervous problems. Salicylic acid contained in violets has a cooling action. Violet flower "tea" assists insomnia and eczema. Use flowers and leaves to make a restorative poultice (see p.125) for cracked nipples; an infusion for a mouthwash for sore gums, and gargle for irritated or inflamed throats; a decoction (see p.123) of the leaves makes a wash for rashes and other skin inflammations, and may be added to creams and lotions (see p.125) for eczema.

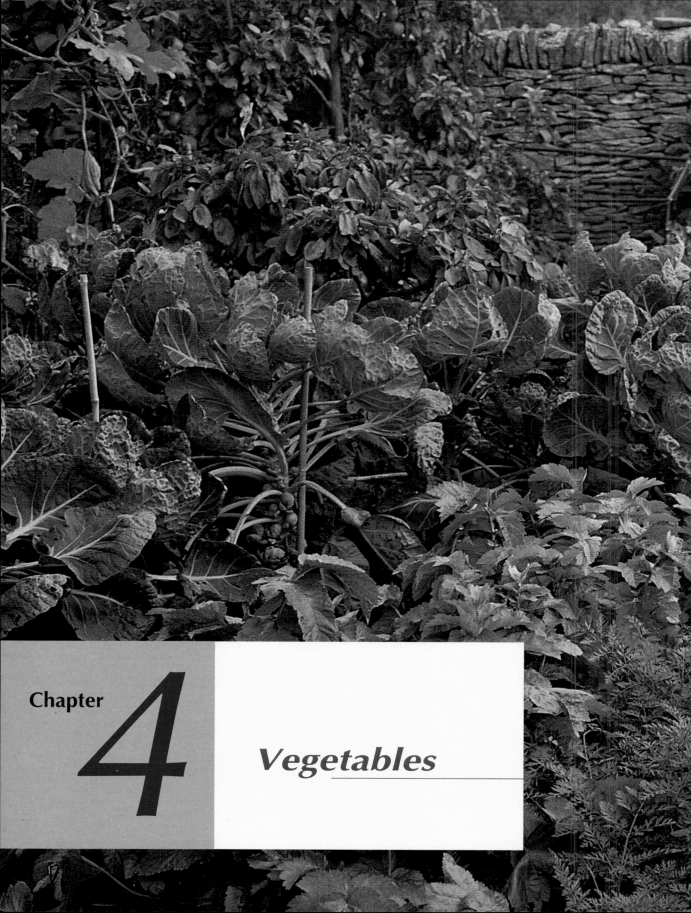

Chapter 4

Vegetables

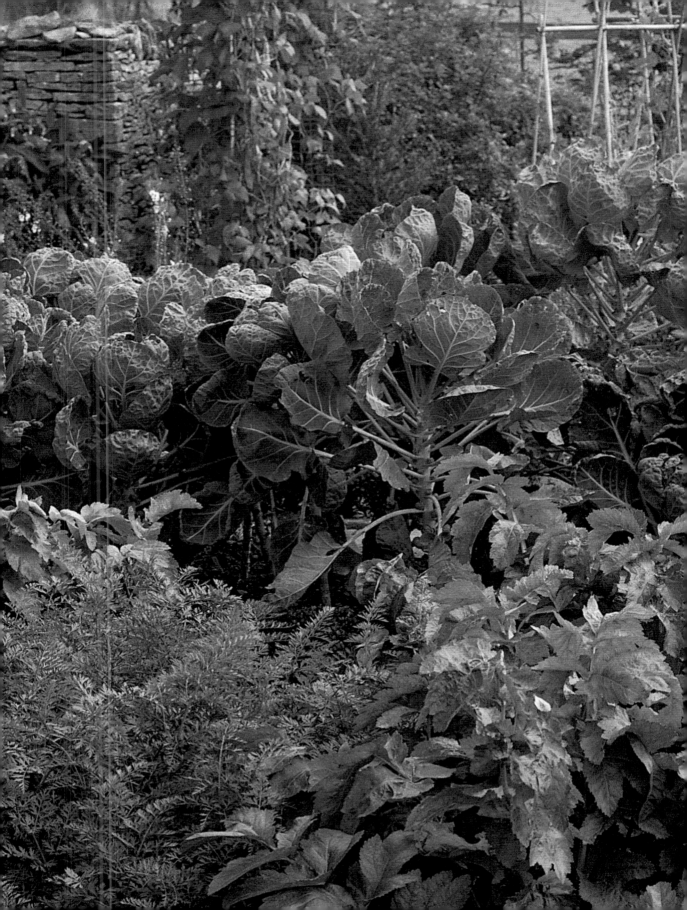

Vegetables

In today's world our immune systems have to deal with diverse pollutants which may weaken our resistance to disease. Over the past half century the body has been asked to cope with far more than it can assimilate. Environmental pollutants at large may be beyond our individual control, but if we follow the path of the Garden Healer, we can be custodians of our own health to a significant degree.

For those with a small garden, the very best antidote to the damaging effects of pollutants and pesticides is to grow your own supply of as many fruits and vegetables as feasibly possible, preferably from assured genetically non-manipulated, organic seeds.

The time has come to re-learn old lessons, still accepted by Native Americans, who do not make a distinction between food and medicine. Food is our preventive medicine. Home-grown produce, the disease deterrent of the past, needs to be reactivated and brought into the present. Even a detoxifying "apple a day..." is a step in the right direction because prevention is better than cure.

The cottage garden, where something of everything grows for consumption or pleasurable use, emerged in Britain after the Black Death (1349-50), when lands not owned by overlords became the property of survivors, and supported the household. The variety of vegetables expanded after the medieval monastic gardens period of cultivated leeks, curly kale, smallage (wild celery) and lettuce as standbys for winter and summer. This continued to be a viable means of vegetable cultivation until the Industrial Revolution. Even today, this type of gardening remains attractive and productive, and eminently suitable for small gardens, often including bee-keeping for the production of healing honey.

RUNNER BEAN FLOWERS

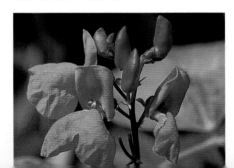

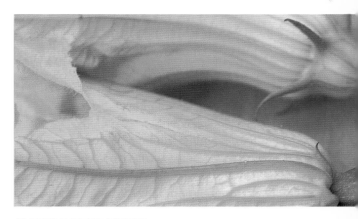

TRAILING MARROW FLOWERS

THE DELIGHTS OF THE VEGETABLE GARDEN
The vegetable garden is enormous fun and a great gourmet experience, for there is history and romance in vegetables. Antiviral garlic (*Allium sativum*) journeyed from Babylon (*c.* 3000 BC) via the Greek and Roman cultures to the garlic festival which takes place annually on the Isle of Wight, Britain. Here, even the beer is garlic-flavoured.

The vegetable garden is a family affair. Children love to plant vital fast-growing radishes (*Raphanus sativus*) and sleep-inducing lettuces (*Lectuca sativa*), and adults enjoy the luxury of diuretic asparagus (*Asparagus officinalis*). Anglo-Saxons knew about curative cabbage, which they called "sproutlake" (curly kale). All the brassicas contain health-giving folates and iron, and coenzymes that speed up biological processes, such as digestion. Broccoli contains the coenzyme Q_{10} – the purple-sprouting variety being the most appealing supplier. The anti-carcinogenic globe artichoke (*Cynara cardunculus* Scolymus Group) is an easy-growing plant equally at home in the flower border, and Jerusalem artichokes are also a wonderful culinary delight.

The preservation of old strains of vegetables is important. Old-fashioned and unusual species provide interest and dietary variety. Celeriac, kohl rabi, Florence fennel, salsify, scorzonera, endive, chicory, Chinese cabbage, winter radish and asparagus peas, add savour to flavour and are affordable when home grown. Using novel solanaceous plants, like red and blue salad potatoes (*Solanum tuberosum*), and yellow cherry tomatoes (*Lycopersicon esculentum*), can make a luncheon or dinner party unique.

As summers grow hotter, and seeds become genetically manipulated, cultivation of home-grown non-genetically engineered gluten-free maize (*Zea mays*) is a conservational option.

Carrot

Carrots have been with us since classical times. They are indigenous to Europe, Africa and Asia, and were naturalized in North America. The roots range from dark red, yellow, orange and purple to white, and are used as animal fodder, food and medicine. In Ireland, where they were very fond of love philtres, carrots were thought to be an aphrodisiac.

Healing Uses: Carrots are highly nutritious, containing vitamins A (ß-carotene), B_1, B_2 and C, and fibre. *D. carota* promotes menstruation, the seeds can treat urine retention and digestive disorders. The oil for massage is antiseptic, a stimulant and liver tonic, vasodilatory and a smooth muscle relaxant. It also aids skin conditions and revitalizes mature complexions. Helpful to indigestion, as well as anaemia and PMS, it detoxifies arthritis and rheumatism. *D. carota* is most beneficial when cooked, and purée can be given to babies with diarrhoea.

Home Uses: Carrot's forte is its supply of contra-cancer ß-carotene, the precursor of vitamin A. It can be juiced and eaten regularly as preventive medicine, and for its contra free-radical input, which adds to the resistant levels of the blood and maintains mucous membranes.

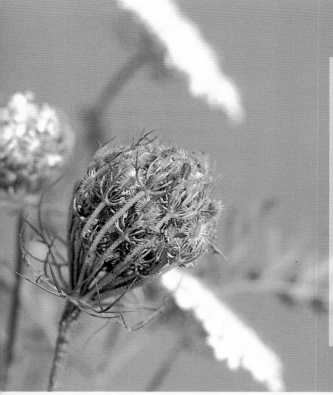

Carrots & Cancer

Carrots have a high β-carotene content and are thus an ideal preventive medicine to counter cancer and other damaging effects of the numerous environmental pollutants in the atmosphere and food chain. Because of organophosphates in commercially grown vegetables, it is necessary to top, tail and peel bought carrots before use, or preferably buy organic ones. Cancer describes any malignant tumour that arises from the abnormal and uncontrolled division of cells, which then invade and destroy the surrounding tissues.

   See pp.132-3.

CARROT (DAUCUS CAROTA)

Globe Artichoke

Artichokes originate from the Mediterranean; both the Greeks and Romans grew them as vegetables. *Cynara* derives from the Greek *kuon*, meaning dog, which refers to the "dog's teeth" resemblance of the purple flower-head bracts. Because of these, the plant is often referred to as the Edible Thistle. Mashed roots of artichoke were used as a deodorant in the 1st century AD.

GLOBE ARTICHOKE (CYNARA CARDUNCULUS SCOLYMUS GROUP)

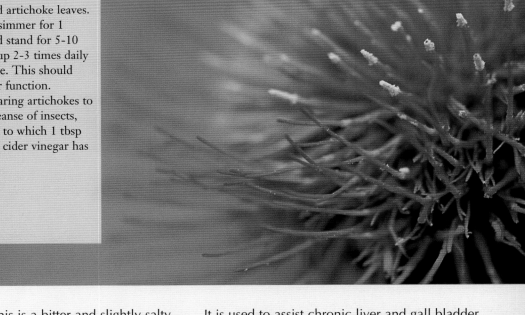

Artichoke Tea

Pour 1 cup of cold water over 1-2 tsp (5-10 ml) dried artichoke leaves. Bring to boil and simmer for 1 minute. Cover and stand for 5-10 minutes. Take 1 cup 2-3 times daily for 1 week or more. This should improve your liver function.

Tips: When preparing artichokes to eat, in order to cleanse of insects, soak in cold water to which 1 tbsp (15 ml) of organic cider vinegar has been added.

 See p.133.

Healing Uses: This is a bitter and slightly salty herb. Artichoke head leaves and/or hearts are an excellent source of folate and potassium. The leaves contain cynarin, a compound proved to enhance liver and gall bladder function. It is a detoxificant which aids the regeneration of liver tissue and stimulates the gall bladder, reduces blood lipids, serum cholesterol and blood sugar.

It is used to assist chronic liver and gall bladder diseases and to treat arteriosclerosis and diabetes.

Home Uses: The globe artichoke is a delicacy which is relatively inexpensive. It can easily be grown and beneficially added to the diet fresh when in season. Traditionally, the unopened flower heads are boiled and eaten hot with melted butter or cold with vinaigrette.

Strawberry

Country dwellers closely guarded the locations of wild strawberries growing in pockets of good soil in secret places. In Britain these fruits have been plundered but they are found more readily in other parts of Europe or the temperate regions of Asia and North America. The good gardener can re-introduce them to the rockery or the patio, or in a large disused stone or porcelain sink.

Healing Uses: All herbalists concede the strawberry is efficacious, using berries, leaves and roots. The antioxidant aromatic berries treat kidney stones and joint pains, having an overall tonic effect. In Ayurvedic medicine the leaves are a "cooling" astringent diuretic. Mildly laxative, they stimulate the liver and the fruit's insoluble fibres improve digestion. The sun-warmed fruits have a great deal of vital energy.

Home Uses: Strawberries are an excellent beauty aid, cleansing inside and out. Ripe cut strawberries help clean discoloured teeth and remove plaque. Make a "tea" with wild strawberry leaves to add minerals to the blood; decocted (see p.123), it is a tonic to strengthen the female reproductive organs. Diabetics can benefit from cultivated strawberry tea (about 5 fresh leaves to 1 cup).

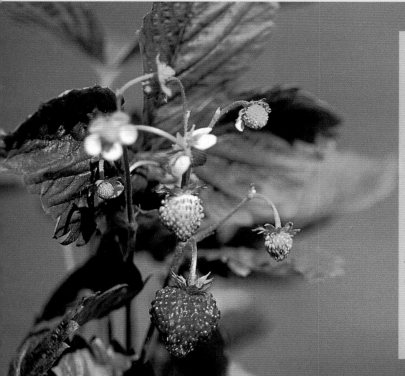

A Luxury Facial

Purchase or pick, clean and dry with kitchen paper ½ pt (¼ lt) prime very ripe strawberries. Mash with fork to manageable pulpy consistency (do not use liquidizer). Apply to cleansed face or other areas and allow to dry for about 15-20 minutes. Rinse off with warm water, followed by cold. For unusually oily skin add the beaten white of an egg to the mixture. For very dry skin drizzle a teaspoonful (5 ml) of avocado or olive oil into mixture before applying.
Tip: Try a patch test before applying to check for allergy.

✳ See p.132.

WILD STRAWBERRY (FRAGARIA VESCA)

Maize

This cultural staple cereal we mostly relate to food is a sacred plant which has been cultivated in the Americas for over 5,500 years. In the Huichol culture of Mexico maize forms the trinity of "creation" with the deer and peyote. In hallucinatory visions the Shamans can see its five colours. Its seeds are donated as offerings, and its shucks are used for making ritual cigarettes.

MAIZE (ZEA MAYS)

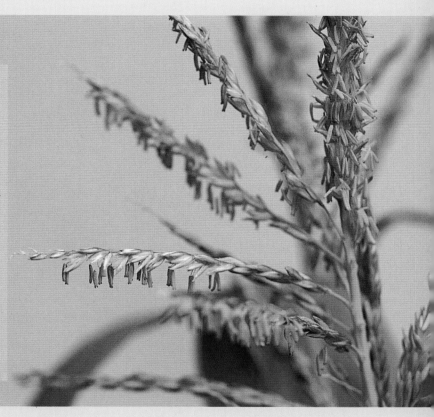

Coeliac Disease

A condition in which the small intestine fails to digest and absorb food, caused by sensitivity of the intestinal lining to the protein gliadin contained in the germ of wheat and rye. This leads to atrophy of the digestive and absorptive cells of the intestine. Maize offers an alternative gluten-free staple diet base for coeliac children.

Tip: Variegated forms of maize – 'Gigantea quadricolour' or 'Gracillima variegata' – are colourful and interesting to dot around the flower border or to grow in clumps.

Healing Uses: Allantoin, the extract from female flowers, was used as a medicine by the Aztecs, and by the Chinese in the 17th century. Allantoin is a diuretic, which lowers blood sugar levels, stimulates bile flow and prevents formation of kidney and bladder stones. It can help in jaundice, hepatitis and cirrhosis.

Home Uses: Steam fresh gluten-free corn-cobs to eat. Use infusions (see p.122) of cornsilk for urinary complaints – cystitis and enuresis in children. Rich in flavonoids, potassium and vitamins C and K, it is especially useful for coeliac disease. An external poultice (see p.125) of corn meal will treat boils and swellings. Cornsilk is a diuretic and tonic, the "tea" of which assists the prostate and male reproductive organs.

Allium

The allium family embraces onions, shallots, garlic, leeks and chives. Ancient in origin and use, onions are derived from the Latin *unio*, meaning "one large pearl" and are a vital base vegetable of cooking and protective dietary food. *A. cepa* (shallot) is a worldwide medicinal vegetable, varying in size, colour and flavour. In China, the shallot is known as "a jewel among vegetables". Purple-flowered Siberian chives (*A. schoenoprasum*) will adorn the garden. The pungent leaves of sand leeks (*A. scorodoprasm*) grow wild by the sea.

Raw Onion Aphrodisiac

An aphrodisiac is a substance which arouses desire. This is usually achieved by scent, human phere-mones or seductive fragrance. Many plants have this reputation, mostly due to their shape and form rather than their content. However, the Breton French "Johnny Onions", who eats raw onions daily, prides himself on his virility.

The lily family, including garlic, is prized in Europe, America, China and India for its effects upon impotence. Success lies in the onion bed through its excellence as a blood cleanser and tonic, ensuring vital good health. Strong blood means sound erections, which are a rush of blood to the reproductive tissue. Raw onions can enhance spermato-genesis and help produce healthy semen through safeguarding and inducing robust health.

Alliums for Thrombosis

Garlic in particular helps to break down fats which make blood platelets sticky and more likely to cause blood clots. Preventive measures to reduce the risk of the disease include a healthy diet (low in cholesterol and saturated fats), moderate consumption of alcohol, keeping fit with regular exercise and not smoking. The four major forms of the disease are: blocked arteries; effects upon the limbs (usually legs); coronary artery blockage, triggering a heart attack; and clots in the blood vessels, which can cause embolism. Thrombophlebitis, which inflames veins closest to the skin, may be associated with varicose veins. Daily intake of alliums is as important to the pregnant mother as to the ageing and elderly.

Tip: Once you cut an onion it will start to absorb germs – so never use a cut onion that has been left out overnight.

Healing Uses: Culinarily fashionable garlic's litany of use is prodigious, but its "heart" is at the core of preventive medicine. Alliums' modest lilies are more usually associated with colds, flu, bronchitis and asthma. Garlic is antibiotic, hypotensive, anti-diabetic and anti-thrombotic, and the oil antiviral. The active compound allicin can kill many kinds of bacteria, fungi and viruses, including *candida* and *salmonella*. Many bacteria still plague modern life in forms of food poisoning or in poor water quality. Onions share much of garlic's prowess and have the added attraction of having many purposes, varieties, and being available all year round.

Home Uses: Following a Mediterranean diet rich in alliums will strengthen the immune system and help treat coughs, colds and stomach ailments. Onions sliced and rubbed on cuts or acne help prevent spread of bacteria. Eat garlic raw or cooked – from winter casseroles to summer salads and infuse in vinegars. Make garlic-honey cough syrup, to apply cosmetically or for herpes. Fill a glass jar with garlic cloves, slowly dripping in honey over two days; then allowing the mixture to macerate in the sun for 2-4 weeks. A quartered onion, one piece placed in each corner of a room, will absorb all malodours quickly. A whole large Spanish onion eaten raw can free one from cold symptoms, if eaten immediately the first symptoms are detected.

Leek Poultice for Skin Boils

For boils reluctant to come to a head, bactericidal leek is an excellent natural cure.
Take a leek, trim the end and cut off the white part. Slice lengthwise into strips and steam. Place lengthwise between two layers of 3-inch (7.5-cm) bandage with spare ends trailing to form a "tie". Test with elbow before applying hot to affected area.
Repeat every hour for three hours to draw the pus to the surface.

✳ See p.132.

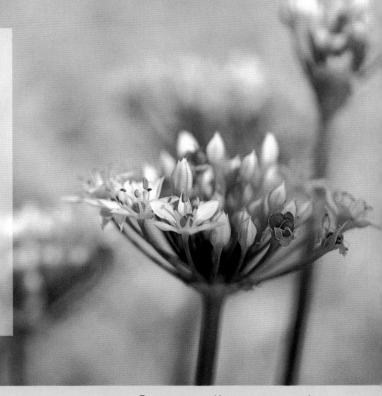

CHINESE CHIVES (ALLIUM TUBEROSUM)

Nasturtium

Nasturtium takes its name from the Greek *tropaion*, meaning trophy, as its flower forms a "helmet" above a leaf "shield". The Spanish conquistadors, who first called it Indian cress, brought it from Peru. This flamboyant Andean herb is a gardener's joy, ornately bright and cheerful, it grows either in clumps, cascades of orange and yellow, or as a climbing vine.

Healing Uses: Whereas watercress (*Nasturtium officinale*) is renowned for its iron content. *Tropaelolum majus* is high in sulphur and contains a glycoside that combines with water to make an antibiotic, used as a disinfectant and to heal wounds. Reputed to retard baldness, *T. majus*'s sulphur is a component of two essential amino acids present in every cell.

Home Uses: Eaten raw the whole plant is antiseptic and a diuretic tonic, helping fight fungal and bacterial infections. Use the leaves, flowers and flower-buds in salads, with cheese and egg dishes and add (at the last moment) to stir-fries to cleanse the blood and benefit digestion. Infuse (see p.122) the flowers to make vinegar and pickle the seeds as capers to go with fish.

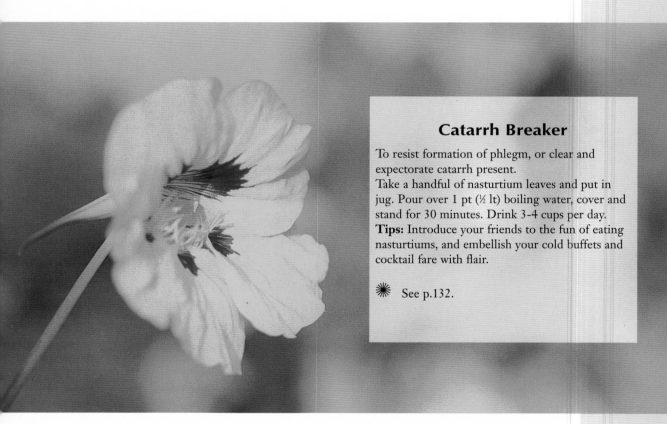

Catarrh Breaker

To resist formation of phlegm, or clear and expectorate catarrh present.
Take a handful of nasturtium leaves and put in jug. Pour over 1 pt (½ lt) boiling water, cover and stand for 30 minutes. Drink 3-4 cups per day.
Tips: Introduce your friends to the fun of eating nasturtiums, and embellish your cold buffets and cocktail fare with flair.

✳ See p.132.

NASTURTIUM (TROPAEOLUM MAJUS)

Asparagus

There is a feeling of sheer opulence about eating fresh asparagus, even from the smallest home-grown raised-bed. Dr Van de Vende (1873-1937) hailed it as an aphrodisiac. Certainly asparagus is upright – a "rod" shape, emerging from the "cup" of its root, two major esoteric symbols of the Egyptians. Ancient Egyptian tomb drawings from *c.* 4000 BC suggest that they used it for urinary and nematocidal applications.

ASPARAGUS (ASPARAGUS OFFICINALIS)

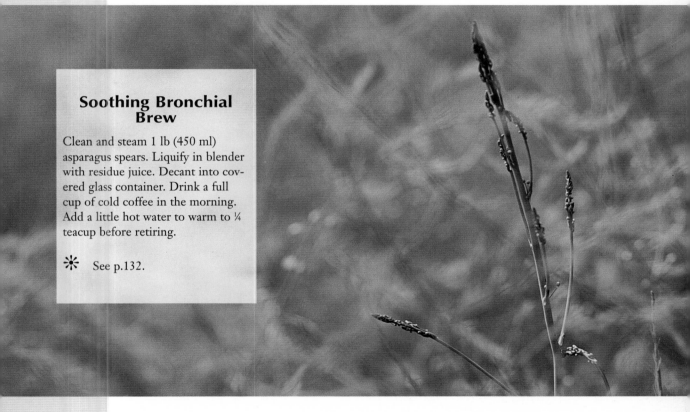

Soothing Bronchial Brew

Clean and steam 1 lb (450 ml) asparagus spears. Liquify in blender with residue juice. Decant into covered glass container. Drink a full cup of cold coffee in the morning. Add a little hot water to warm to ¼ teacup before retiring.

✳ See p.132.

Healing Uses: The spears are nutritious, rich in folate, containing vitamins C and E, plus anti-carcinogenic ß-carotene. Fresh asparagus is an excellent detoxificant for rheumatism. It is diuretic, laxative and a cardiac tonic, and expels waste products accumulated in the joints via the urine. The Oriental maritime *A. cochinchinensis* will soothe inflammation, control coughs and stimulate salivation.

Home Uses: Mainly used to treat cystitis, pyelitis, kidney disease, rheumatism and gout, asparagus is a seasonal vegetable that deserves to be eaten for general health, if not for libido and pleasure alone. As a detoxificant steam young fresh spears or make a soup or purée. Alternatively, make an infusion/"tea" (see p.122) as a diuretic drink from the shoots and/or the fern-like leaves when the plant is going to seed.

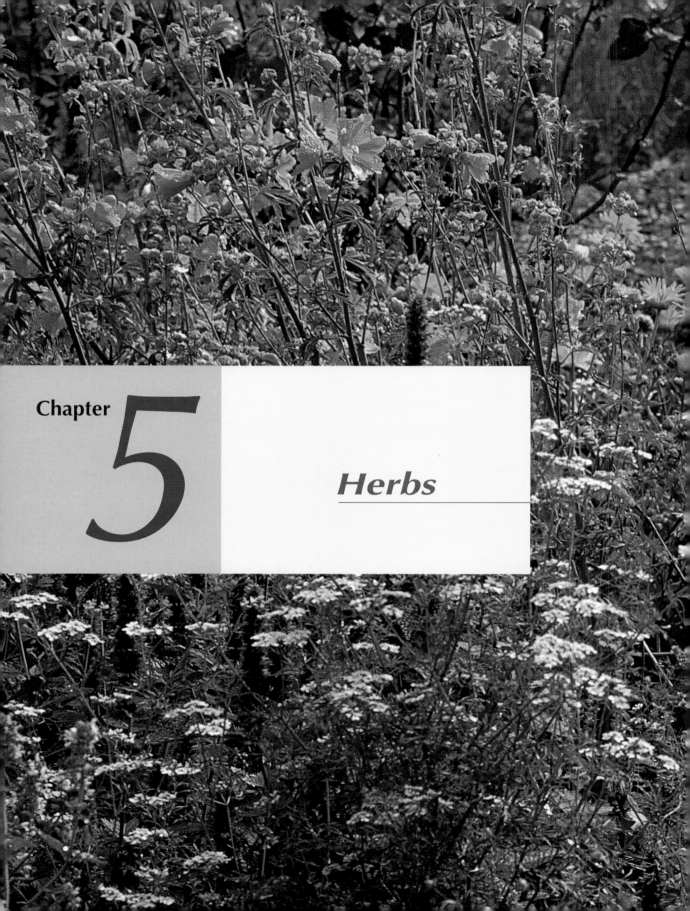

Chapter

5

Herbs

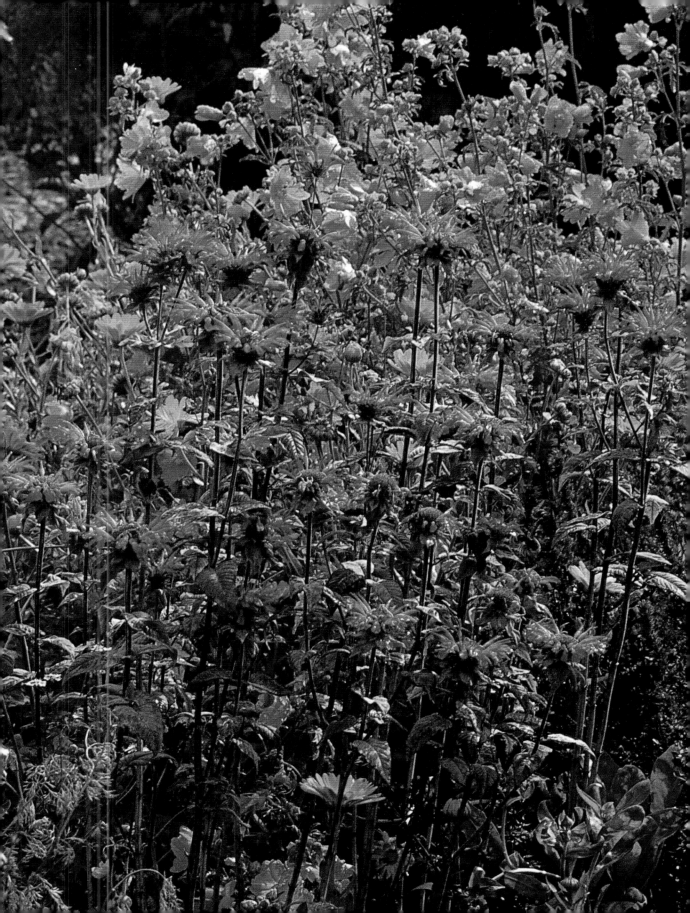

Herbs

The garden offers us a unique source of inspiration in the form of culinary, medicinal and enjoyable herbs. Nowhere else can be found, concentrated in one place, the immense wealth of raw materials for healing and improving our quality of life.

The majority of people are familiar with the culinary use of parsley, thyme and sage, which rank among the most common herbs. For instance, parsley is known as an accompaniment to fish; thyme is used to scent honey; and sage is familiar as a key ingredient of stuffing, all of which help us to celebrate the landmarks of the year.

Whether Christmas and Easter in Europe, Thanksgiving in America, or Chinese New Year, herbs are an integral part of our culinary traditions and religions, automatically fulfilling an important medicinal role through diet and nutrition.

Herbalism offers an enormous number of healing options in many different forms – from teas, infusions, concoctions, decoctions, compresses and poultices to extracts, powders, potions and pills.

Herbs, with few exceptions, also have their active principles replicated or synthesized for use in allopathic medicine. These same herbs produce the essential oils used in aromatherapy. In this treatment their essence is absorbed into the body's bloodstream through the skin, and their perfumes enter the brain through the olfactory system, healing mind and body simultaneously.

In the arena of vibrational medicine, plant and flower essences also come directly from herbs to heal the emotions. In homoeopathy , the power of a herbal essence is captured and used by reducing it down to a "blueprint" that is passed to the body through ingestion.

GINSENG

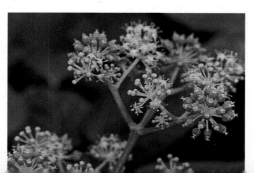

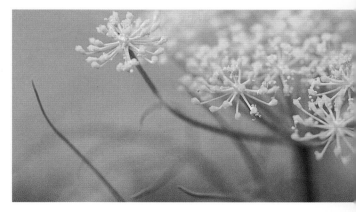

FENNEL

ORIENTAL HERBS

The Garden Healer need not be deterred from growing exotic remedial herbs. Ginseng (*Panax ginseng*), from the Greek *pan* meaning "all" and *akos* ("cure"), and the Chinese *gin* ("man") and *seng* ("essence"), has been used as a tonic in the Orient for at least 5,000 years. In the reign of Britain's Charles II it was valued at thrice its weight in silver. Later found growing in Canada and described by botanist Joseph François Lafitau, *Panax trifolius* was used widely by the local Iroquois as a stimulant tonic, especially for treating extreme exhaustion. Subsequently, *Panax quinquefolius* was found in Pennsylvania.

A hardy perennial, requiring protection from frost in winter and from humidity during the growing season, ginseng propagated from seed is a long-term investment ready to harvest when 6-7 years old. Meanwhile, those less patient, happy to mobilize pots (inside and out), can take a much shorter route to romantic rhizomes, and dabble in ginger (*Zingiber officinale*) to titillate their tastebuds, assist stomach upsets, liverish digestion and winter colds.

EUROPEAN HERBS

Fennel (*Foeniculum vulgare*) was sacred to the Anglo-Saxons, and grown in 812 AD in the imperial gardens of Charlemagne. The entire anise-flavoured plant is restorative. It was the food of lusty gladiators, and aided Roman matrons with obesity. It is now used in moderation for oedema and cellulite. Dill (*Anethum graveolens*) is good for hiccoughs and, being rich in mineral salts, aids a salt-free diet – as does borage (*Borago officinalis*). Infused chervil (*Anthriscus cerefolium*), a traditional French *fine herbe,* will stimulate digestion, and caraway seeds (*Carum carvi*), popular in Germany and the Middle East, will sweeten the breath and relieve flatulence.

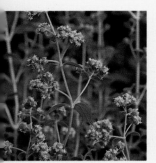

SWEET MARJORAM

"And this delightful Herb
whose tender Green
Fledges the River's Lip
on which we lean -
Ah, lean upon it lightly!
For who knows
From what once Lovely Lip
it springs unseen!"
Rubayat (c. 1100)
by Omar Khayyam

Many simple herbs like yarrow (*Achillea millefolium*) make remedial "teas". Lemon balm (*Melissa officinalis*) alleviates bronchial catarrh, feverish colds and headaches; bergamot (*Monarda didyma*) helps nausea, menstrual pain and insomnia; and sweet marjoram (*Origanum majorana*) used as a flower-top "tea", or decocted for a bath, is a relaxant. The slightly aromatic golden rod (*Solidago virgaurea*) is a sudorific antiseptic.

VIRTUOUS WILD HERBS

Herbs of infinite variety and use grow everywhere. If not content to let wonderful weeds and wildflowers hold sway in the flower borders, be adventurous when siting those plants commonly styled "herbs". For in truth the assertive herbs, "garden thugs", such as mint, if securely bucketed, will transport diversity to any part of the garden.

Garlic and chives (*Allium spp.*) that deter greenfly are welcome elsewhere. Nasturtiums can glow beneath apple trees and repel aphids. Ground elder and bindweed are not happy in the company of French marigolds (*Tagetes patula*), the scent of which does battle with tomato white fly.

It is useful to have a bed, however small, of common culinary herbs near to the kitchen. Bear in mind when planting that herb gardens seldom resemble the cooled and forced displays to be seen at flower shows. Herbs have tall spikes and spirals that lean over threateningly, before falling about the place like drunken sailors, scattering their seeds in all directions.

Low-lying plants can become moth-eaten in appearance, in need of a judicious trimming to remedy their unsightliness. Remember, herbs were pagan catholics of unbridled habit long before Christianity, and many remain free spirits.

CHERVIL

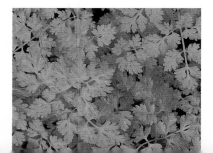

Comfrey

Comfrey, the Roman's "knitbone", derives from the Greek *symphyo*, "make grow together", and *phyton* "plant". Employed in Ayurvedic medicine, it is a Russo-European perennial fodder crop, as well as a nutritive human tonic with more leaf protein than any other vegetable. A triumph of nature's victuals, it contains vitamins A, C and B_{12}, calcium, potassium, phosphorus and starch.

Healing Uses: Comfrey is a miracle herb credited with a multitude of cures. The leaf and roots contain allantoin, which encourages cell division, and predisposes its ability to heal external wounds and ulcers. The "tea" helps internal ulcers, reducing inflammation of the stomach lining, and coughs. Throughout history, it has proved the best herb for mending broken bones.
Home Uses: Recent research has indicated that internal use of comfrey is not advisable. However, used as an external macerated oil (see p.124), compresses, washes, poultices (see p.125) and a simple ointment, it is an invaluable healer. Fresh leaf compresses and poultices reduce swelling of sprains, and aid sores, burns and cuts. Infusions (see p.122) added to baths and lotions soften the skin.

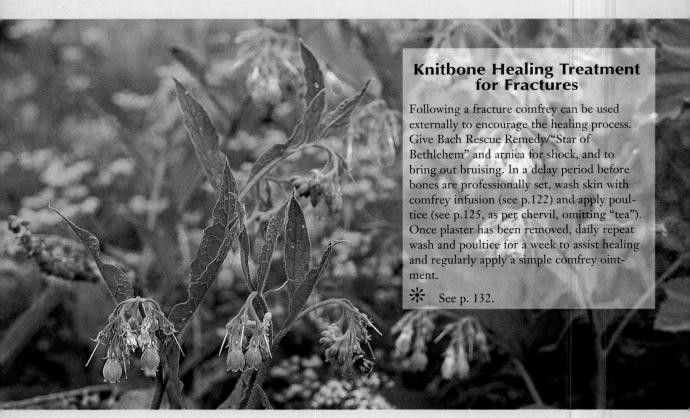

Knitbone Healing Treatment for Fractures

Following a fracture comfrey can be used externally to encourage the healing process. Give Bach Rescue Remedy/"Star of Bethlehem" and arnica for shock, and to bring out bruising. In a delay period before bones are professionally set, wash skin with comfrey infusion (see p.122) and apply poultice (see p.125, as per chervil, omitting "tea"). Once plaster has been removed, daily repeat wash and poultice for a week to assist healing and regularly apply a simple comfrey ointment.

✳ See p. 132.

COMFREY (SYMPHYTUM OFFICINALE)

Coriander

Coriander (from the Greek *koris* for "bug") is named after the bug-like odour of its flowers. It was cultivated as a medicinal herb by the Ancient Egyptians, Chinese, Indians and Greeks. An emblem of immortality, this biblical culinary herb is used in Jewish Passover food. It has been part of popular culinary tradition since its introduction to Europe by the Romans.

CORIANDER (CORIANDRUM SATIVUM)

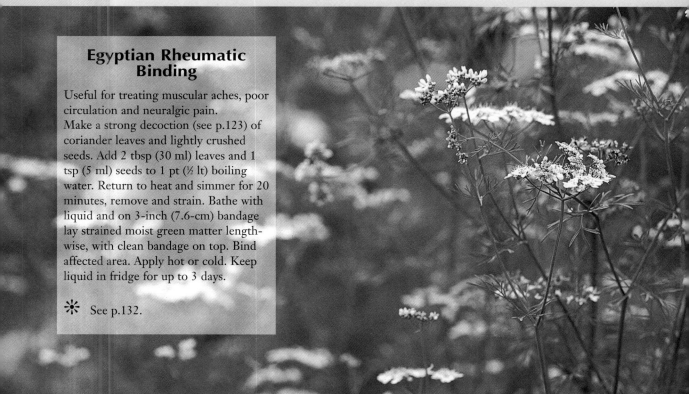

Egyptian Rheumatic Binding

Useful for treating muscular aches, poor circulation and neuralgic pain.
Make a strong decoction (see p.123) of coriander leaves and lightly crushed seeds. Add 2 tbsp (30 ml) leaves and 1 tsp (5 ml) seeds to 1 pt (½ lt) boiling water. Return to heat and simmer for 20 minutes, remove and strain. Bathe with liquid and on 3-inch (7.6-cm) bandage lay strained moist green matter lengthwise, with clean bandage on top. Bind affected area. Apply hot or cold. Keep liquid in fridge for up to 3 days.

✳ See p.132.

Healing Uses: Coriander seeds used in India, often together with cumin and fennel, still retain their same digestive use today. Especially for diarrhoea and dysentery, promoting the assimilation of other herbs for blood circulation and digestion.
Home Uses: Press and extract from the leaves the juice to treat allergies, hay fever and skin rashes, (take 1 tsp (5 ml), 3 times per day) and apply it externally for itching and inflammation. Chew the seeds or infuse (see p.122) as a "tea" for a digestive tonic or mild sedative. Eat the leaves in stews, salads and sauces; the seeds in curry, soups and vegetable dishes; the stem with beans and in soups; and steam the fresh root. The oil is good for muscular aches, poor circulation, neuralgic pain and nervous exhaustion.

Lovage

Early spring lovage in medieval times was an aphrodisiac known by the French as *luvesche* ("loveache"), and employed in potions to cure heartache. Alpine lovage (*Levisticum officinale*) grew in Ligurian Italy in great abundance. The juice and smell of lovage was once believed injurious to the eyes. A traditional and modern herb, lovage continues to be used in herbal love baths.

Healing Uses: A bitter-sweet sedative, lovage is pungent and aromatic. An infusion (see p.122) will reduce fevers, relax spasms and aid indigestion, colic and flatulence, and stimulate appetite. It is employed for painful menstruation and to assist slow labour.

Home Uses: Use lovage seeds like pepper for seasoning or add to creamed potatoes or to rice, or sprinkle on salads. The footsore and weary may lay leaves in boots and shoes. Add leaves to stocks, stews, and eat raw in salads. Massage with lovage essential oil is a good rheumatic detoxificant, helping relieve fluid retention and poor circulation. Add it to a cream (max. 2½%, 1 drop per 2 ml) for sore feet and foot problems associated with gouty conditions.

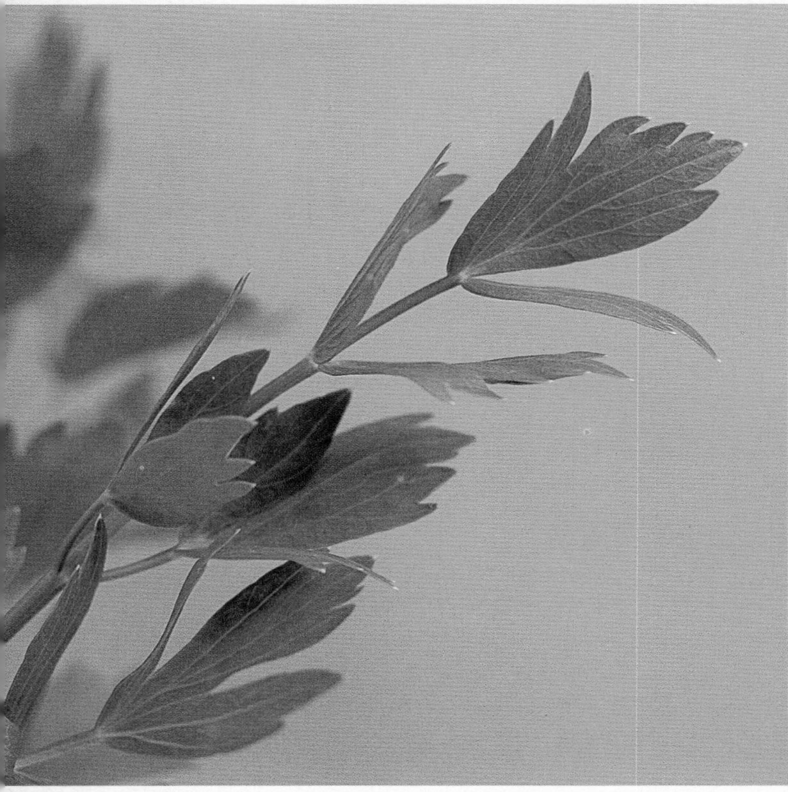

Lovage for Sore Throats

Lovage relieves the small aphthous ulcers associated with sore throats. They occur singly or in groups in the mouth as white or red spots. Make lovage leaf infusion (see p.122) and swill mouth and gargle regularly for 3-4 days to a week, until the condition has abated.

❊ See p.132.

LOVAGE (LEVISTICUM OFFICINALE)

Tarragon

The worldwide horticultural offspring of Greek goddess Artemisia are a vast clan. Its name comes from the French *estragon* or *herbe au dragon* (*L. dracunculus*), and tarragon is a "dragon" of the Orient and Occident, with its fiery taste and serpentine roots. Spanish tarragon retains its vinegary character from Arabic Moorish influence, whilst coarser progeny grow prolifically throughout Russia.

TARRAGON (ARTEMISIA DRACUNCULUS)

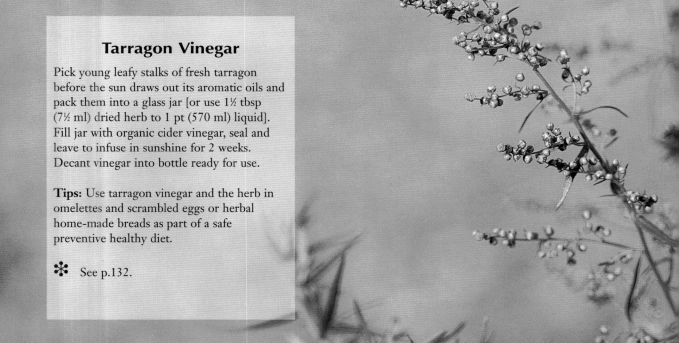

Tarragon Vinegar

Pick young leafy stalks of fresh tarragon before the sun draws out its aromatic oils and pack them into a glass jar [or use 1½ tbsp (7½ ml) dried herb to 1 pt (570 ml) liquid]. Fill jar with organic cider vinegar, seal and leave to infuse in sunshine for 2 weeks. Decant vinegar into bottle ready for use.

Tips: Use tarragon vinegar and the herb in omelettes and scrambled eggs or herbal home-made breads as part of a safe preventive healthy diet.

✳ See p.132.

Healing Uses: Tarragon is well beloved by French and Spanish cuisine alike. Its leaves, rich in iodine and mineral salts, contain vitamins A and C and have the ability to alleviate toothache and rheumatism (which can follow over-indulgence of rich foods). In warmer climes it is used to treat threadworms in children. Its cousins wormwood and mugwort are less sanguine and should be treated with caution.

Home Uses: Growth of this benefactor to the head, heart and liver, is to be encouraged, for its spicy leaves do well in salads, sauces and soups. This *fine herbe* accompanies chervil, chives and parsley, goes with egg-dishes, fish, poultry, game, liver and kidneys. An infused "tea" (see p.122) of the leaves is digestive and a general tonic.

Parsley

Mountain parsley (*Petroselenum crispum*) was Ancient Egyptian medicine's contra-diuretic. It was highly esteemed by the Ancient Greeks, crowning victors of the Isthmian games. Mediterranean peoples still use fern-leaved parsley and flat parsley (*P.c.* var. *neapolitanum*) as culinary medicine. Hamburg parsley (*P.c.* var. *tuberosum*) is an interesting vegetable cooked like carrots or grated raw in salads.

Healing Uses: All parsleys are antiseptic culinary herbs containing vitamins A, B and C, iron and flavonoids, and are antioxidant. Parsley is used as an emmenagogue in Ayurvedic medicine to promote menstruation and clear blood clots. Roots, leaves and seeds contain apiol, beneficial in the treatment of jaundice.

Home Uses: Use parsley infusion (see p.122) as a hair tonic and conditioner. Either a mild digestive "tea" of the leaves (*P. crispum*), or a stronger "tea" of the seeds assists rheumatism, gall bladder function and cystitis. Eat raw as a garnish or use in dishes of *fines herbes* and *bouquet garnis*. The leaves are highly nutritious and may be used as a mineral supplement.

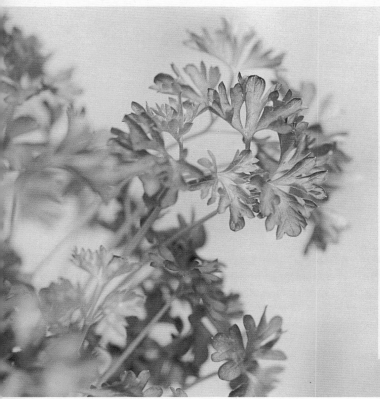

Parsley Jelly for Digestive Circulation

Clean a large bunch of parsley and place in saucepan with sufficient water to cover. Add lemon peel and simmer gently for an hour. Strain liquid into glass bowl, adding juice of 3 lemons. Measure, allowing ½ cup each honey and sugar to each cup liquid. Return to pan and bring to boil. Mix in proprietary fruit pectin with warm liquid. Cool and pour into mini-moulds or glass jars. Cover, seal, label and date. Store in cool place or refrigerate. This goes well with white meat or fish.
(Adaptation from an R. Hemphill recipe in *Herbs of all Seasons*).

❋ ❀ See pp.132-3.

PARSLEY (PETROSELINUM CRISPUM)

Thyme

The Greek gods gave thyme as a gift to poets and physicians, and to the bees that still make the famously delicious Grecian honey of the Hymettos hills. *Thymus* means "courage", and was bathed in by Roman soldiery for vigour. This esoteric herb of the Middle Ages provides enormous healing strength and vitality, and possesses a powerful reviving perfume.

COMMON THYME (THYMUS VULGARIS)

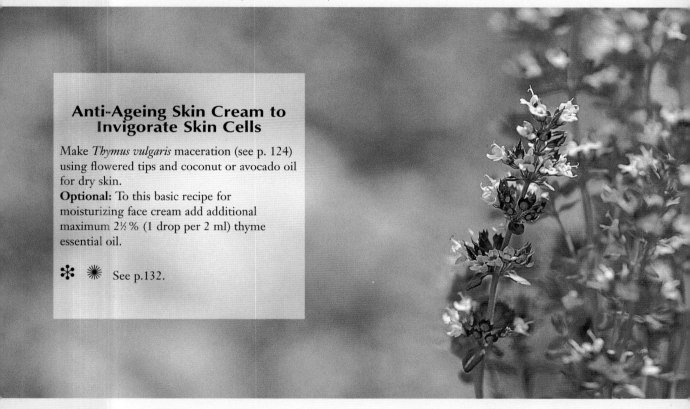

Anti-Ageing Skin Cream to Invigorate Skin Cells

Make *Thymus vulgaris* maceration (see p. 124) using flowered tips and coconut or avocado oil for dry skin.

Optional: To this basic recipe for moisturizing face cream add additional maximum 2½% (1 drop per 2 ml) thyme essential oil.

✽ ✳ See p.132.

Healing Uses: A powerful herb for overcoming infections and respiratory illnesses such as flu and bronchitis. It inhibits growth of germs and decreases thickness of bronchial secretions, whilst stimulating the digestion. It has an invigorating tonic physical effect, yet is sedative upon the nerves, sharing the same name "thymus" as the gland crucial to the immune system.

Home Uses: Infusions (see p.122) may be used for hangovers. A syrup made with honey assists convulsive coughs, cold symptoms and sore throats. A maceration (see p.124) or massage with essential oil brings relief from sciatica and rheumatic pains. Add lemon-scented thyme to refreshing hair rinses. Thyme's culinary abilities are as many as its varieties, from *bouquet garnis* to stocks, marinades, stuffings, sauces, soups and dishes cooked in white wine.

Sage

The diversity of *Salvia's* colours and foliage is a gardener's salvation. A sacred herb of Ancient Roman and Greek ceremonies, sage is "wise" and is derived from the Latin *salvere* "to be in good health, cure or save". The Chinese and Persians valued it for longevity, considering it thrice more precious than China tea. In Roman times, gardeners were advised not to use iron tools, as iron salts are incompatible with sage.

Healing Uses: Aromatic sage breaks down fatty foods and orchestrates other flavours. Its antiseptic, anti-fungal and astringent properties aid mouth and gum problems. It is a stimulating tonic, encouraging the flow of irregular menstruation, good for stress and shock, and useful for menopausal problems and to reduce lactation.

Home Uses: Scatter leaves in linen to discourage insects. Sage leaf "tea" will arrest mild diarrhoea, promote menstrual blood flow or, after eating, stimulate digestion; it has a calming nervine effect. The gardener and cook will appreciate purple sage (*S. officinalis* Purpurascens Group) and balsamic Spanish sage (*S. lavandulifolia*), red and gold prostrate sage, plus the euphoric scent of clary sage (*S. sclarea*). The essential oil is good for muscular pains. Try pineapple sage in late summer in butters, jellies and compotes.

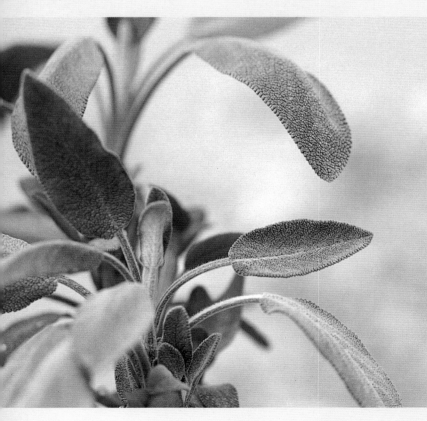

A Sagacious Infusion for Gingivitis

Take 1 tsp (5 ml) dried sage leaves or 1 tbsp (15 ml) fresh, and pour over ½ pt (¼ lt) boiling water; cover and stand for 10-15 minutes. Swill and gargle mixture in mouth and throat. Use frequently to subdue inflammation associated with gingivitis and to strengthen gums. Do not swallow.

✳ ✳ See p.132.

COMMON SAGE (SALVIA OFFICINALIS)

Mint/Spearmint

Perfume and medicine were synonymous when Egyptian mint was an ingredient of *kyphi*, the world-renowned Egyptian incense. A biblical herb, the Pharisees collected it with dill and cumin as tithes, and it was used to decorate the synagogues of the Hebrews. Mint, a potential garden thug, still shows its rapacious masculine character in its growth, and feminine constitution in its use.

SPEARMINT (MENTHA SPICATA)

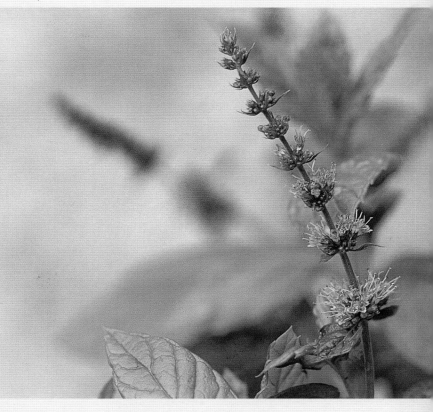

Flatulence & Nausea Tea

To 1 cup boiling water add 1 tsp (5 ml) dried or 2 tsp (10 ml) fresh mint (*M. spicata*). Cover and stand for 10 minutes. Then drink hot after eating to disperse wind or nausea.

Tip: Grow spearmint and peppermint near roses to deter aphids. Essential oil of *M. spicata* will help fatigue and boost the immune system against infection. Add to cream for acne and congested skin.

✻ ✻ ✤ See pp.132-3.

Healing Uses: Mint is versatile with invigorating qualities. Externally, it is aromatic and cooling in hot weather and its multiple uses range from culinary and household to aromatic and medicinal. Mint tea is a traditional antiseptic Bedouin beverage, assisting indigestion, nausea and headaches, biliousness and PMS.

Home Uses: Macerate (see p.124) carminative creeping pennyroyal (*M. pulegium*) in oil to apply externally for chest infections. Peppermint (*M. x piperita*) "tea" helps respiratory ailments. Infuse (see p.122) fragrant eau-de-Cologne mint (*M. x piperita* 'citrata') or ginger (*M. x p.* 'Variegata') for scented hair rinses to stimulate the scalp. Use *M. spicata* for inhalations to loosen and disperse catarrh. Use applemint (*M. suaveolens*) in desserts and jellies. Mint is the best addition to lamb and dark chocolate sauce.

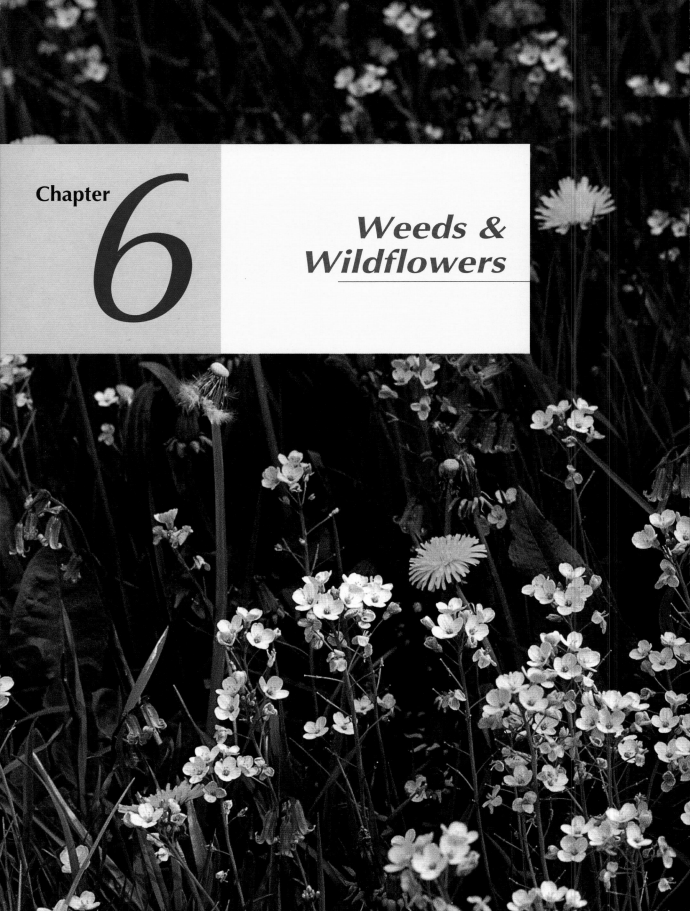

Chapter

6

*Weeds &
Wildflowers*

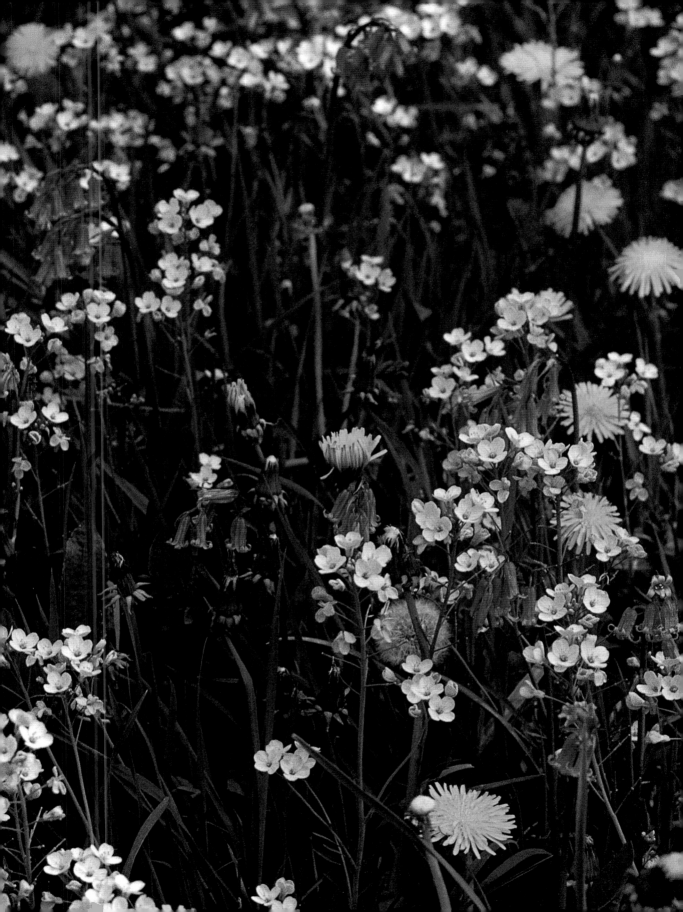

Weeds & Wildflowers

One definition of a weed is "any plant growing where it is not wanted". Another is "plants we don't yet know the use of". Every precious cultivar and remedial herb was once wild. In that context a self-seeded lupin flourishing in the middle of a gravel driveway is a weed. Conversely, some of the most gardener-unfriendly plants are indeed wonderful weeds.

A prime example is couchgrass (*Elymus repens*), which has been an important world-wide medicinal herb, recorded since the 1st century AD by Dioscorides. Male gardeners might like to know that, in common with horsetail (*Equisetum spp.*), its invasive silica-rich rhizomes are used in preparations for prostatic treatment, in particular for enlarged prostate. Romanies also used a cold-water couchgrass decoction for temperature reduction and gall stones, which will also serve as a garden spray for mildew and fungus.

Couchgrass – the unwanted "vandal" of vanity lawns and well-groomed borders – has also been cultivated for use as a nutrient foodstuff.

THE VERSATILITY OF WEEDS

The Garden Healer will find that erstwhile weeds are very versatile everywhere. *Avena sativa*, the oats and groats of Scotland (packed with protein, starch, minerals and vitamin E), started out in life as a wild weed. In peaty soils the heather and ling (*Calluna vulgaris*) that scents the air and furnishes bees with nectar is found on heath and moorlands around the globe, and gives remedies for nervous exhaustion and insomnia. Ditch-happy wild celery (*Apium graveolens*), rich in vitamins and mineral salts, makes a leafy tonic infusion and its seeds ease flatulence. Nightshade (*Atropa bella-donna*), a poisonous plant, made history via atropine, and preceded anaesthetic as

CHICORY

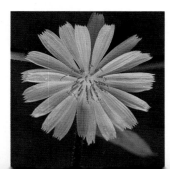

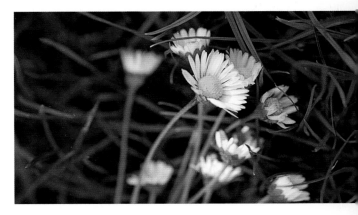

DAISY

"sorcerer's pomade". Another member of the family, *Solanum dulcamara* or "bittersweet", treats chronic rheumatism. We relish its many solanaceous cousins like aubergine, potatoes and tomatoes, for a multitude of culinary uses in the kitchen.

Potage herbs of the past and condiments of the present are marvellous weeds. Wild horse-radish (*Armoracia rusticana*) has an extra bite to its flavour, cleanses the blood and stimulates digestion. Mustard seed (*Brassica juncea* and *B. nigra*) contributed condiments and spices to the Orient long before the Romans brought them through Europe to produce pain-relieving, antibiotic poultices and plasters for rheumatism, muscular strains, and footbaths for the common cold.

Sorrel is so good, picked when young and eaten raw, or cooked like spinach, that the French decided to cultivate it, yet it is more often ignored as a mere weed instead of a

gourmet treat. Skirret (*Sium sisarum*), a Chinese pot herb is said to be "the most delicious of root vegetables".

It takes but a spark of inspiration to use the legions of dandelions (*Taraxacum officinale*) and burdock (*Arctium lappa*) for greens, coffee, wine and beer; nettles (*Urtica dioica*) for spinach, soup and beer; bistort (*Persicaria bistorta*) for Easter pudding; and Sweet Cicely (*Myrrhis odorata*) for French fritters. Even ground elder or "gout weed" (*Aegopodium podagraria*) may be eaten as a vegetable.

Herbs like chickweed (*Stellaria media*), astringent common daisy leaves (*Bellis perennis*), or sophisticated blanched chicory (*Cichorium intybus*) can be used in salads. Summer puddings, jams and wines can be made from the elder (*Sambucus nigra*), and blackberry (*Rubus fruticosus*). Other sweets of the wild include sloe gin (*Prunus spinosa*), wild mints (*Mentha spp.*), hazel nuts (*Corylus avel-*

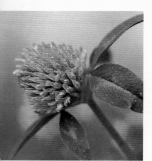

RED CLOVER

"Trample under foot,
The daisy lives and strikes its root
Into the lap of time: centuries may come
And pass away into the silent tomb,
And still the child,
hid in the womb of time,
Shall smile and pluck them, when this
simple rhyme shall be forgotten."
Collected Poems by **John Clare**
(1793-1864)

lana) and haw jelly (*Crataegus monogyna*). All are remedial herbs, or garnishes and flavourings with medicinal qualities.

Many colonial herbs were once European weeds. Native Americans smoke bearberry leaves (*Arctostaphylos uva-ursi*) with tobacco and women use it for cystitis. Aromatic alecost (*Tanacetum balsamita*), used in cuisine, cosmetics and medicine, and "cherished for its sweete flowers and leaves", was brought to America by the Puritans.

There are aggravating weeds that cling to our clothes when busy in the garden, such as sweet woodruff (*Galium odoratum*) and cursed ground ivy (*Glechoma hederacea*), used by early Saxons to clarify and improve the flavour of their beers. Tenacious cleavers (*Galium aparine*) lowers blood pressure and is used in the treatment of ME (myalgic encephalomyelitis), hepatitis, benign breast tumours and cysts. White horehound (*Marrubium vulgare*) is another common multi-purpose weed, and attracts bees into the garden.

Scented weeds such as melilot or yellow sweet clover (*Melilotus officinalis*), spread their perfume to bees from Asia to Canada. Red or purple clover (*Trifolium pratense*) is the most important forage crop of Northern Europe. It is a herb, which, in common with violets, can be cosmetic, eaten in salads or used for a fragrant wine. Spring provides us with the sunshine yellow of sweet-smelling cowslips and pale primroses (*Primula veris* and *P. vulgaris* respectively). With their sedative and expectorant properties they relieve spasms and relax mind and body.

Among the wonderful wildflowers, the most revered for emotional ties is the fiery-red, sleep-inducing poppy, contrasting with the intense blue eyes of cornflowers (*Centaurea cyanus*), whose florets aid corneal ulcers. The sacred greater celandine (*Chelidonium majus*), or "Alchemists' gold", is used by swallows to open the eyes of their young with its sap, and is also employed externally for human cataract. Legend and myth tell how these wonderful jewels dropped from heaven. They are plants of the gods which help compose the mind and give us flower essences to help our psyche and emotions.

Perhaps ambitions for manicured lawns and weed-free borders have driven out the wonder and delectation missing in a world of high technology. Or, again, we may have lost the art to distinguish between weeds, wildflowers and herbs, which in truth are all one and made of the same star-stuff as ourselves. The Garden Healer may live to see the meeting point of the influences of Ancient Greek astronomer Hipparchus (*c.* 146-120 BC), who catalogued the stars and gave understanding of the seasons, and Hippocrates (*c.* 460-377 BC), the Father of Medicine – for many of their secrets are encoded in the garden disguised as weeds and wildflowers.

CORNFLOWER

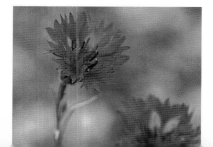

Ivy

A symbol of immortality, and sacred to Egyptian Osiris, god of abundance and fertility, evergreen ivy has been with us since the 7th century BC. Obesity is not a thing of the past and ladies who have cellulite in the 1990s have stolen a march on their forebears with the use of this admirable herb for external beauty preparations to help treat the condition.

Healing Uses: *The Leech Book of Bald* (900 AD) gave a recipe for tender ivy twigs boiled in butter to make a salve for sunburn, especially of the face. Highlanders of Scotland took Irish ivy (*Hedera hibernica spp.*) foot corn salve to America and also used *H. hibernica* to make a weak internal decoction (5 leaves to 1 cup) for swollen glands.

Home Uses: In our modern world it is better to employ ivy externally. Use a strong decoction (see p.123) for an eczema "coolant"; add to cream for cellulite massage; prepare poultices (see p.125) for pustules and on-site skin problems such as boils; use to eradicate corns formed by inverted pyramidal skin layers, causing pain.

Ivy & Cellulite

Cellulite is not recognized medically. It is characterized by dimpled, orange-peel-like skin, particularly of the thighs' "jodhpurs", and buttocks. Thought to be due to accumulation of toxins in the fatty tissues, individuals do not need to be overweight to have the condition. Fundamental to its removal is a healthy diet, low in fat, sugar, salt, tea, coffee, alcohol, processed foods and additives. Plenty of fresh fruit and vegetables and 2 litres of pure water per day will reduce toxicity. Anti-cellulite preparations will only work if there is a review of diet. Ivy, with its reductive action, is an excellent aid for counteracting cellulite.
See p.128 for ivy massage cream.

✳ See p.132.

COMMON IVY (HEDERA HELIX)

Cowslip

Dedicated to the Norse goddess Freya, the cowslip is the "true primrose" and is known throughout Christian Europe as "St. Peter's Keys". Its flowering heralds summer weather. Almost picked to extinction in Britain during the first quarter of this century, the cowslip is a wildflower that deserves the attention of gardeners to encourage its growth and preservation.

COWSLIP (PRIMULA VERIS)

Cowslip Tonic Wine

3 lb (1½ kg) loaf sugar
1 gallon (4½ lt) spring water
2 oranges (grated rind and juice)
1 lemon (grated rind and juice)
1 gallon (4½ lt) cowslip flowers
2 tbsp (30 ml) brewer's yeast
½ pt (¼ lt) brandy (optional)

Place water and sugar in cauldron, bring to boil, stir and skim carefully. Put rinds and juices of fruits in big pan. Add boiling sugared water mixture and stir well. Allow to cool to tepid, then add cowslip flowers (de-stalked and cleansed) and yeast. Stir thoroughly, cover with muslin, and allow to stand for 48 hrs. Add brandy. Turn into clean cask, bung and leave for 2 months. Draw off, strain, bottle and store in cool place.

  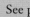 See pp.132-3.

Healing Uses: Cowslip's distinctive fresh fragrance is embodied in the wine. High in flavonoids, it is a tonic for the debilitated (drink one glassful per day before retiring). Floral infusions (see p.122) reduce fever and are anti-inflammatory. The roots have long been employed in treating arthritis. The tincture and "tea" of woodland primrose (*Primula vulgaris*) flowers are mostly used for nervous disorders and as a poultice (see p.125) to heal wounds.

Home Uses: Make a "tea" of the flowers to ease headaches. The flavonoids are anti-inflammatory and antispasmodic, inhibiting histamine release, and antioxidant. Macerate (see p.124) flowers in oil or make an ointment for sunburn. Eat *P. vulgaris* flowers raw in salads or boil as a vegetable.

Chickweed

Chickweed is perhaps the most universal weed in the world. The star-studded plant has followed humans wherever they settled and was used as "greens" for domestic fowl. In Britain during Elizabethan times (1533-1603), this bird food was called "passerina" and fed to caged song-birds such as linnets.

Healing Uses: Apart from important vitamin C, chickweed contains potash (potassium) salts and rutin. It is an alternative "tea" for rheumatism and bronchitis. Decoctions are used for constipation internally, piles and sores externally, and wound-healing cold compresses. It is a nutritive herb of Ayurvedic medicine, a moistening expectorant and external healer.

Home Uses: Excellent for summer and winter salads, or steamed as a vegetable. A fresh-leaved poultice (see p.125) will relieve inflammation and ulcerations, or alternatively bathe areas with a chickweed decoction (see p.123). Cooling chickweed healing ointment can be used to calm itchy skin irritations.

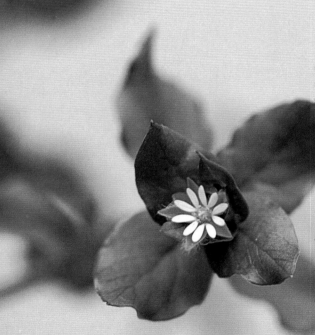

Chickweed Ointment

Cut handful chickweed, mix with handful dried rose petals and boil in grape juice (1½ fl oz/40 ml) until reduced by one quarter and strain.
1 tbsp (15 ml) beeswax
1 tbsp (15 ml) lanolin
2 tbsp (30 ml) chickweed decoction (see p.123)
10 drops lavender essential oil
1 tsp (5 ml) glycerine
1 tbsp (15 ml) cocoa butter
1½ tbsp (22½ ml) calendula oil
¼ tsp (1¼ ml) borax
Melt beeswax in bain-marie, separately lanolin and cocoa butter, add and stir in latter to beeswax. Warm calendula oil and glycerine and slowly stir into mixture. Dissolve borax into chickweed decoction and continue stirring until thick. Add lavender oil when cool. Decant, close, label and date.

✳ ✳ ✳ See p.132.

CHICKWEED (STELLARIA MEDIA)

Horsetail

Horsetail is a hardy, spore-bearing, plant that bestrides the world, except Australia, and is virtually unchanged since forming whole forests in Palaeozoic times. High in silica, its abrasive properties were used from medieval times as flails, scouring pads and metal cleaners. Some horsetails have minute deposits of gold which miners use as visual clues for locating potential sites.

FIELD HORSETAIL (EQUISETUM ARVENSE)

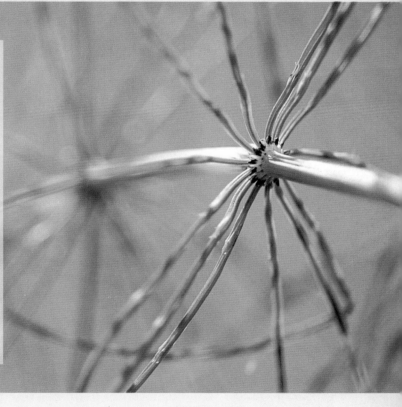

The Prostate Gland

This gland may become enlarged in elderly men, obstructing the neck of the bladder, impairing urination. The bladder then dilates, increasing pressure on the kidneys. If the swelling obstructs the bladder outlet, urination is difficult, frequent, urgent and painful. Usual treatment is the removal of the gland, but horsetail infusions and decoctions can be used – with qualified care – as a means of relieving symptoms of an enlarged gland.
See p. 126 for Gardener's Nail Treatment.

✳ ✳ ✳ See p.132-3.

Healing Uses: Horsetail is the sole known source of organic soluble silica available to humans. Bitter-sweet *E. hyemale* is used in Chinese medicine for eye inflammations, and in Ayurvedic medicine for urinary tract complaints, fractures and venereal disease. Restricted to short-term use, field horsetail is used internally for prostate problems, usually in conjunction with *Hydrangea arborescens* or other demulcent herbs, or for kidney ailments when boiled in wine.

Home Uses: The most practical usage of *E. arvense* is for brittle or splitting nails, not uncommon in earth-delving gardeners. Horsetail is useful to have on hand to staunch external wounds and nosebleeds, as it is an excellent clotting agent. A decoction (see p.123) added to a bath will assist slow-healing fractures.

Dandelion

Arab physician Avicenna first recorded the therapeutic usage of the dandelion. The "Lions' Teeth" leaves (*dents de lion*) sustained the inhabitants of Menorca through a famine, and Canadians and British alike enjoy its beer. Food of Hecate, the golden sun-rayed wonder weed has ethereal fairy-clocks which delight children even in the grimiest cities.

Healing Uses: Dandelion leaves, roots and young tops are high in vitamins A (ß-carotene), C and niacin B complex. They contain potassium, calcium and one and a half times more iron than spinach. A diuretic power-house of nutrients, dandelion cleanses the blood, treats skin and kidney disorders and fluid retention.

Home Uses: Use young leaves for diuretic "tea", and in nutritious salads with mildly laxative bitters of grated or chopped raw root. The leaves, high in potassium, will replace any lost during diuresis. Steam, like spinach, as a vegetable. Grind the dried and roasted root as a decaffeinated coffee substitute. Decoct (see p.123) the flowers for a cosmetic wash. Use the leaves in facial steams as a spring tonic.

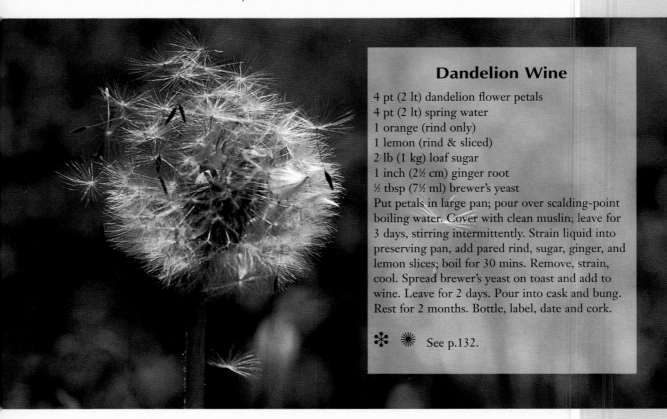

Dandelion Wine

4 pt (2 lt) dandelion flower petals
4 pt (2 lt) spring water
1 orange (rind only)
1 lemon (rind & sliced)
2 lb (1 kg) loaf sugar
1 inch (2½ cm) ginger root
½ tbsp (7½ ml) brewer's yeast

Put petals in large pan; pour over scalding-point boiling water. Cover with clean muslin; leave for 3 days, stirring intermittently. Strain liquid into preserving pan, add pared rind, sugar, ginger, and lemon slices; boil for 30 mins. Remove, strain, cool. Spread brewer's yeast on toast and add to wine. Leave for 2 days. Pour into cask and bung. Rest for 2 months. Bottle, label, date and cork.

✳ ✱ See p.132.

DANDELION (TARAXACUM OFFICINALE)

Nettles

Stinging nettles, renowned for their burning pricks, have been used in medicine since ancient times. Less favoured by gardeners than silvered-leaf lamiums, the white deadnettle (*Lamium album*) takes its name from *lamium*, Greek for "gullet", referring to the nectared "throat" of its flowers. A one-time vegetable in France, *L. album* are called "dead" as they do not sting, unlike their lookalike counterparts, stinging nettles.

NETTLE (*URTICA DIOICA*)

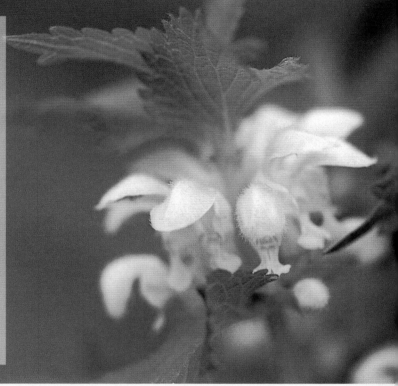

Anaemia

Due to its high iron content *U. dioica* makes an excellent "tea" to treat anaemia. Take 1 tsp (5 ml) of dried herb (2 tsp (10 ml) of fresh) to 1 cup of water, 2-3 times a day. Anaemia is a reduction in the quantity of the oxygen-carrying pigment haemoglobin in the blood. The main symptoms include excessive tiredness, breathlessness at exercise, and poor resistance to infection. It can be due to blood loss through haemorrhage from an accident, chronic bleeding, iron deficiency, destruction or the impaired production of red blood cells. Treatment depends on the cause, which must be professionally diagnosed and treated.

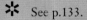 See p.133.

Healing Uses: *L. album* is used in "teas" for bladder disorders, the female reproductive system, and prostate problems. *U. dioica* is rich in iron, vitamins A and C, and vital salts and minerals. It is an excellent medicinal food eaten young in spring, where the vitamin C content ensures iron absorption. An astringent, terrific tonic, diuretic and detoxificant, it controls uterine bleeding and assists in reducing high blood pressure and sugar levels. *U. dioica* aids arthritis, rheumatism, eczema, and in particular anaemia caused by excessive menstruation.

Home Uses: Use *L. album* or *U. dioica* in decoctions to condition hair. Use *U. dioica* for washes, infusions (see p.122), decoctions, and compresses (see p.123) to treat the complaints in healing uses. For anaemia, young leaves can be eaten as a vegetable or soup, or drunk as a "tea".

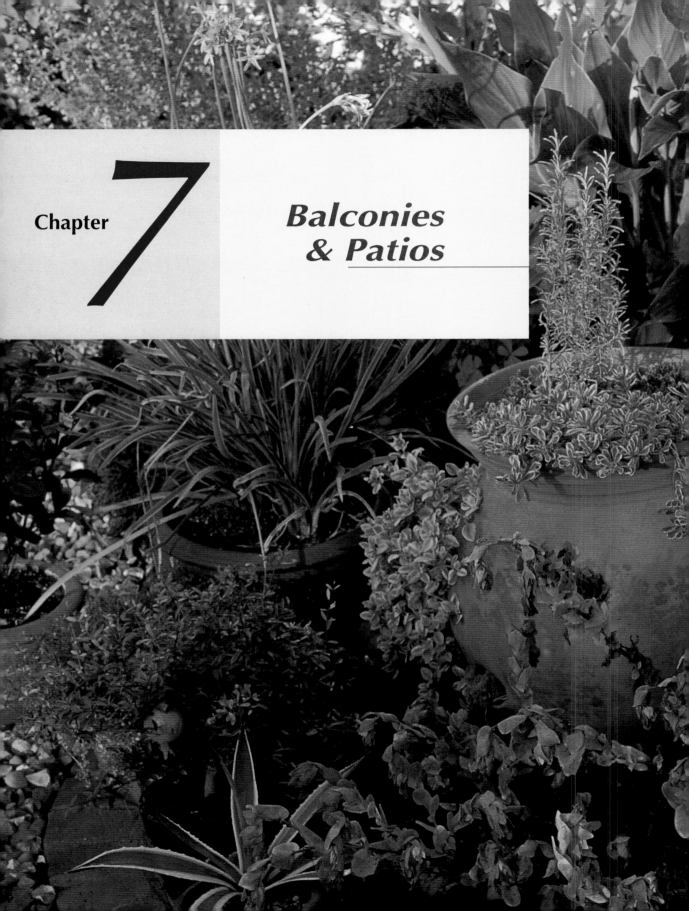

Chapter

7

Balconies
& Patios

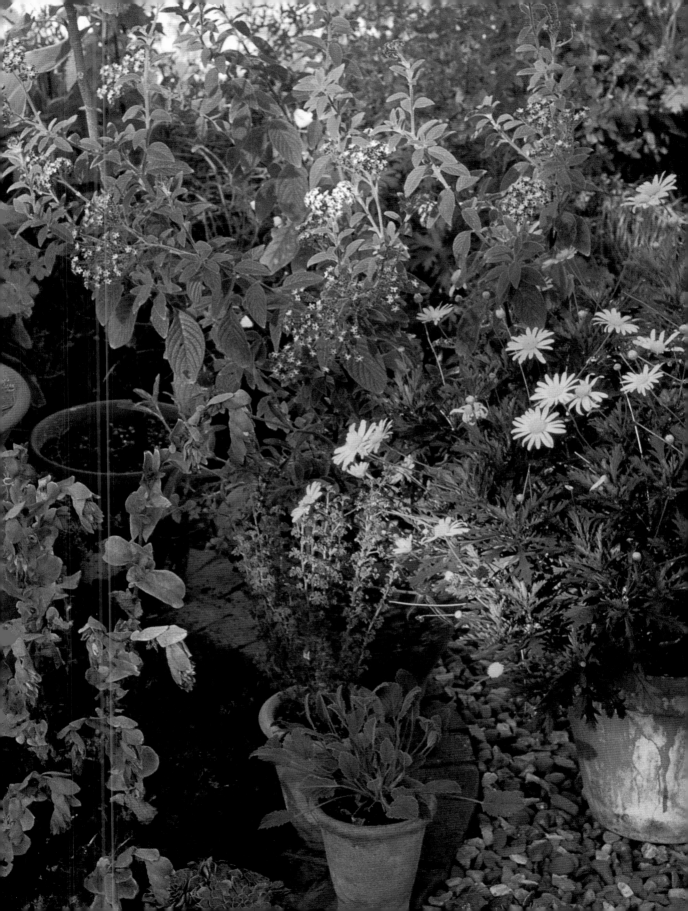

Balconies & patios

We have come a long way since nature was sole architect of the universe, and humans were cave-dwellers surrounded by space and all things natural. Nature was our role model, giving us the wheel contained within a tree's trunk, and mechanization was born. Trees with touching canopies inspired the spiritual ideology of great cathedrals of worship for religion. As we gained deeper comprehension of mathematics, we honed our emulative skills, copying the wildlife that lives in every garden. Civilizations like those of the Mayans and Egyptians used geometry in architectural design which had more in common with insects such as bees.

Eventually, humans began to take architecture out of its original context, away from its natural environment and the flow of nature. We created dwellings from a succession of geometric boxes, then furnished the exteriors with plants, gradually turning ourselves into urban residents, pushing the boundaries of contact with nature further away.

The rapid acceleration of development and progress in the past half century has led us to lose touch with the balance of our environment. Modern housing estates, with little but tree-lined avenues and patches of grass, destroyed many habitats of wild flowers and herbs. Yet even older community parks can still be a source of wild material, as are disused railway lines and neglected canals. Undaunted, practical gardeners have turned waste and unwanted civic land into town allotments. Garden Healers have never given up creating a portion of paradise on earth for their own.

THE TOWN-DWELLERS' PATIO
In warmer parts of Europe a subtle Arab influence trickled down through urban lifestyle.

NARCISSUS TAZETTA

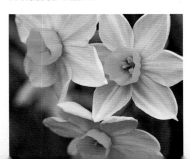

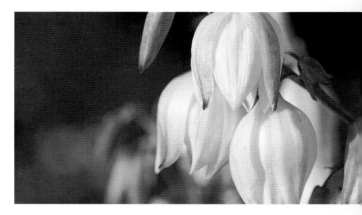

YUCCA

The Spanish Moorish influence of the Alhambra Palace, in Granada, found its common counterpart in the building of water sites central to the house. Potted plants lined walkways, such as the famous Street of Flames, in Cordoba, where Spanish pride combines with fiery flowers to engulf every wall, lending artistry and fragrance to everyday living, and easy access to culinary and remedial herbs. From this was born the town-dwellers' patio.

The fundamental decoration of patios can reflect the roof of the sky, on blue walls clad with red, or green and white ivies, and picturesque climbing flowers. Use a contemplative maze of pebbles and coloured paving for floors, and water features set into walls, or central to an architectural sculpture of claypots, wood, stone, metal, tiles or glass. Furnish it with a disused wheelbarrow filled with flowers, or cocktail trolley with holes for potted plants. A patio will not accommodate a forest, nor a balcony the Hanging Gardens of Babylon. But we can share in the enjoyment of small trees in tubs, from living columns of junipers (*Juniperus communis*), upright or bossed, and canopied spring cherry (*Prunus spp.*), to exotic blooms of the magnolia (*Magnolia spp.*) for cookery and hedonism.

To delight the eye and sense of smell in spring, plant troughs of warm-scented wallflowers (*Erysimum cheiri*), colourful edible tulips (*Tulipa*), pansies (*Viola*) and daffodils and poetic narcissus (*Narcissus pseudonarcissus* and *N. poeticus*). In large flowering pots plant aesthetic exotic white-flowering yucca (*Yucca gloriola*); sunny-scented cistus (*Cistus landanifer*); multi-scented geraniums (*Pelargonium spp.*) and herbal tormentil (*Potentilla erecta*).

There are a wealth of options on which to draw to compose a remedial planter or culinary-remedial window box. Try tomato-

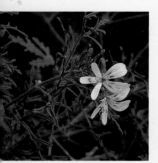

SCENTED PELARGONIUM

"They have been the delight of many a man in whom the love of nature was inborn... but whose means were spare, whose leisure time was scant, and whose advantages in pure air and light and garden space were poor and cramped."
Introduction by Rev. Francis Horner to *Hardy Florists Flowers* **by James Douglas**

loving basils (*Ocimum basilicum*), lemon-scented (*O. b.* var. *citriodorum*) or the purple variety (*O. b.* var. *purpurescans*); parsleys, curly parsley (*Petroselinum crispum*) and flat-leaved Italian parsley (*P. c.* var. *neapolitanum*); oriental coriander (*Coriandrum sativum*); and creeping thyme (*Thymus serpyllum*), white-flowering *T. s.* 'Snowdrift', crimson *T. s.* var. *coccineus*, and golden lemon *T.* x *citriodorus* 'Aureus'. For colour, plant sages – balsamic (*Salvia lavandulifolia*), red and variegated (*S. officinalis* Purpurascens Group and *S.o.* 'Tricolor'), and golden (*S. o.* 'Icterina').

CREATING A PATIO
Let your imagination have full rein, using seasonal sense and gardening acumen to produce masterpieces of display and ingenuity. Venture fruits and vegetables in a tub, or a floral food pyramid to decorate your patio and your dining table with living ornaments to tempt the tastebuds. Grow plants in earthenware pots, one within the other – base pot,

trailing nasturtiums; middle pot, pansies and violas; and top pot, scented geraniums. Or build a scented spring-flower pyramid of base pot, daffodils and narcissus; middle pot, wall-flowers; top pot, snow-drops and sweet violets, to caress the spirit and clear the mind.

Hanging baskets can furnish patio walls or do wonders for the entrance and exit to a home. Whilst providing scent and colour they can also be your victual salad baskets.

A Garden Healer can as well live in a high-rise block of apartments as on a country estate. Nature is eclectic. The town and city dweller with a patio, balcony, or even a humble window box can grow at least some of their own fresh food and medicine. In truth, there are often greater feelings of achievement and pleasure taken in creating something made from next to nothing.

THE PLEASURES OF A GARDEN

A fragment of paradise that pleases the senses and can contribute to our welfare is an opportunity that awaits everyone. Careful seasonal management can produce inventive diversity. As the English Edwardian plant collector Reginald Farrer said: "But a little garden, the littler the better, is your richest chance of happiness and success."

As we move towards the third millennium, we cannot hope to live as simply and gloriously as "the lilies of the field" of biblical times, but everyone is able to improve the quality of life. Organic gardening – growing plants for our pleasure, sustenance, and remedial to our health – is a very real way of making an important individual offering to redress this imbalance for ourselves and for the world. Gardening is for every age, kind and type of person. All who garden can be secure in the knowledge that they are doing some good.

SNOWDROPS

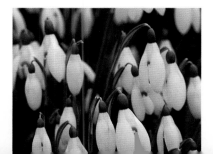

Scented Summer Troughs

Colour and scent brighten our moods and emotional lives. Night-scented stocks planted in a window-box, reconstituted stone or clay cast troughs, with a skirting of pretty pansies and/or the brilliant colours of Livingstone daisies, will reward the eye by day and the nose at night. Set upon an outer windowsill, their welcome fragrance will waft into a room on the evening breeze. Taller tobacco flowers are most effective when bunched together in a tub or in an old sink seated on a balcony or in a patio at ground level.

Scented Summer Troughs

Night-scented stocks
(*Matthiola longipetala* subsp. *bicornis*);
Tobacco flowers
(*Nicotiana affinis* and *N.* x *sanderae*);
Pansies & violas
(*Viola* x *wittrockiana* & *Viola spp.*);
Livingstone daisies
(*Dorotheanthus bellidiformis* syn. *Mesembryanthemum criniflorum*)

Tobacco Flowers

Nicotiana was named in 1560 after the French ambassador to Portugal, Jean Nicot, and was first inhaled as snuff. It was grown in gardens of the Iberian Peninsula for its curative powers, before it was established as "tobacco" in the late Elizabethan period in the City of London. The white starred flowers of evening-scented tobacco have a sweet perfume, and *N. suaveolens*, the annual of Australia, is richly night-fragrant.

Livingstone Daisies

Many gloriously coloured glaucous species of *Mesembryanthemum ciriniflorum* (*Aizoaceae*) grow all over the world, from beside Spanish roads to among the rocky crevices of South Africa. In temperate climates the sheer joy of the equatorial strident flush of colours catches the eye and transports the imagination to islands of paradise. The African Dutch Hottentot explorers discovered this colourful little plant which comes in bright shades of red, pink, yellow or white, the flowers only opening up when the sun shines.

Hungary Water

1 gal (4½ lt) grape spirit
2 oz (60 ml) essential oil of rosemary
1 oz (30 ml) essential oil of balm
1 oz (30 g) lemon peel
1/16 oz (2 ml) essential oil of mint
1 pt (½ lt) each extract of rose and orange-flower, or 2 pt (1 lt) rose water
Blend together and bottle.
This recipe was given to Queen Elizabeth of Hungary in 1370 by a hermit. She kept her beauty late in life through use of it, seducing and marrying the King of Poland at age 72.
From *Scented Flora of the World* by Roy Genders.

Healing and Home Uses: It is not yet known to what extent the scents of common culinary herbs contribute to health. Locked into their essential oils are fragrances that when released uplift the heart, balance the emotions and compose the mind. Aromatherapy has shown that essential oils work simultaneously on physical, psychological and spiritual levels.

There are hidden benefits in the sight of colourful flowers, such as vibrant mesembry-anthemums, and by inhalation of the diverse semi- and demi-tones of plants' and flowers' odiferous molecules we sense as beautiful perfumes. For instance, the scent of mint and rosemary is appetizing and also promotes mental clarity.

The Garden Healer naturally benefits greatly from this combination of enveloping colour and scent. Taste and smell are physically so closely linked that flowers like lavender, violets and roses have flavours similar to their aromas.

The sense of achievement a gardener can feel from nurturing a coloured symphony of scent from seed is sublime – like a living miracle. For within a tiny seed is contained all these sensory aspects of an organic creation of fact and fantasy that can be housed in something as simple as a summer trough.

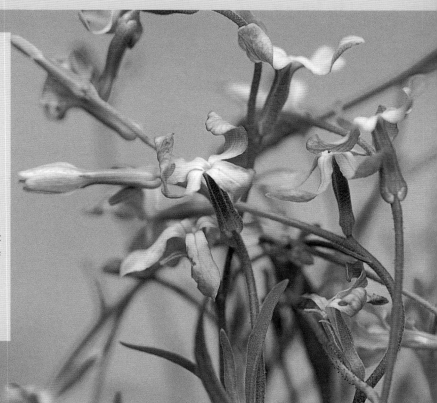

Night-Scented Stocks

There are stocks for all seasons with heady and heavenly scents and softly muted hues. Originally, only the white and the dame's violet (*Hesperis matronalis*) or purple stocks grew, and all were used in conserves, cordials and "eaten now and then". The romantic native night-scented stocks of Spain and Greece have insignificant flowerets varying in colour from white to brown, which store their sublime odorous treasure until nightfall.

NICOTIANA TABACUM (SOLANACEAE)

Skin & Hair Care Planters

For the seasonal plantation of remedial flowers, use elegant indoor planters on external windowsills, balconies and in patios in summer, as well as mixed planting direct into window-boxes. Plant marigolds and chamomile densely in an old bucket, wooden or galvanized; providing drainage holes and a base of "crocks" (fragments of china), with a layer of gravel on top. Copy the common Greek habit of planting houseleeks in urns aloft or at ground level for a good display of this first-aid herb.

Skin & Hair Care Planters

Marigold *(Calendula officinalis)*;

Roman & German chamomile

**(Chamaemelum nobile & Matricaria recutita)*;

Houseleek *(Sempervivum tectorum)*

Chamomile to Calm the Nerves

The central nervous system is responsible for the integration of all nervous activities. Chamomile relieves nervous tension and all stress-related conditions, many of which are the root cause of other nervous disorders encountered through the pressures of modern living. The volatile essential oil of Roman chamomile is predominantly sedative, where-as German chamomile is a stimulant of leucocyte production. The osmotic nature of skin, allows the remedial power of oils applied to the body in aromatherapy to enter the blood- stream. At the same time the odiferous molecules of chamomile penetrate the limbic system of the brain via inhalation of their scent, thereby having a direct calming effect on the central nervous system.

Chamomile Shine for Fair Hair

To make a strong infusion of chamomile (see p.122) add 2 tbsp chamomile flowers (dried) to 1 pt (½ lt) spring water for blonde hair and use regularly. For fair hair that has grown dingy make a decoction (see p.123), boil for 20 minutes using equal amounts of herb and water, to restore the "fairness" and shine. **Tips:** Use the infusion as a wash for sunburnt skin and the decoction for cool compresses for damaged skin or for minor burns. For chamomile skin treat-ment add 2½% (1 drop per 2 ml) chamomile essential oil to a base cream or lotion.

Healing Calendula

Marigold is antiseptic, antiviral and bacteri-cidal, good for healing chapped and cracked hands of gardeners. A quick alternative to making a cream is to add *Calendula officinalis* essential oil at 2½% (1 drop per 2 ml) to a bought prepared base cream.

Healing Uses: Marigold, chamomile and houseleek are all practical herbs that have multi-use for skin care. Today's proprietary preparations containing such herbs vary little from folk recipes, secure in the knowledge that the original cures have proved safe for millennia. The use of houseleek has simply been superseded by aloe in popularity.

Home Uses: Marigold flower infusion (see p.122) makes a good cold compress (see p.123) or binding to heal inflammation of the skin and wounds. A wash of the "tea" is soothing for conjunctivitis. Calendula cream made from marigold flowers can incorporate flower essence or essential oil for the face, and a stronger infusion of petals will tone blemished skin and act as a hair rinse for redheads. From a culinary point of view, flower petals may be used like saffron added to rice, fish soup, soft cheeses, butter, omelettes, cakes, biscuits and sweet breads. The leaves can also be sprinkled in salads.

German "blue" chamomile applied in massage or in a skin lotion is an excellent analgesic and anti-inflammatory oil for acne, burns, boils, cuts, chilblains, eczema, insect bites and rashes. It also makes a good antiseptic ointment and is fungicidal. Its relative *Chamaemelum nobile* has similar properties. The familiar houseleek is a ready-to-hand gardener's aloe for minor burns, wasp and nettle stings, cuts and insect bites.

Calendula Cream

1 tbsp (15 ml) beeswax
1 tbsp (15 ml) lanolin
1 tbsp (15 ml) cocoa butter
1½ tbsp (22 ml) calendula oil (macerated in sweet almond oil, see p.124)
1 tsp (5 ml) glycerine
¼ tsp (1¼ ml) borax
2 tbsp (30 ml) marigold infusion (see p.122)
10 drops calendula essential oil

This is an excellent remedy for nappy rash, cradle cap and sore nipples.

Melt beeswax in bain-marie. Separately melt lanolin and cocoa butter and mix into beeswax. Warm macerated calendula oil and glycerine and slowly stir into bain-marie. Dissolve borax in warm calendula infusion and add to main mixture, stirring well until thick. Cool, mix in essential oil and decant into sterilized glass jars. Cover, label and keep for up to 6 months.

 See p.133.

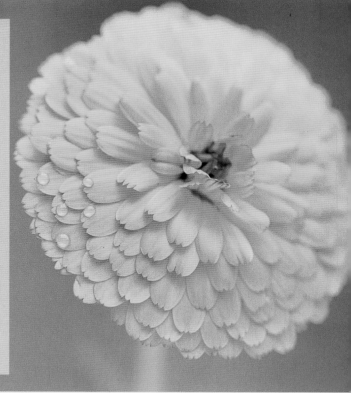

POT MARIGOLD (CALENDULA OFFICINALIS)

Fruit & Vegetables in a Tub

South American potatoes came to England in 1585 and tomatoes in 1596. Offshoots of the vast and decorative *Solanaceae* family, both became important to our staple diet. Potatoes are excellent for cleansing the earth before planting other crops. Tomatoes may be bottled, puréed or sun-dried, or if unripe, made into chutney. Beans can be salted or frozen for winter, whilst marrows and pumpkins are perfect for dry storage.

Fruit & Vegetables in a Tub

Tomatoes & Potatoes
(Lycopersicon esculentum & Solanum tuberosum);

Wild Strawberries *(Fragaria vesca)*;

Climbing haricot beans *(Phaseolus vulgaris)*;

Trailing marrows/Courgettes
(Cucurbita pepo)

Solanum for Weight Watchers

Tomatoes are low in calories. Yellow tomatoes have a higher sugar content than red ones. Eat steamed, boiled or baked potatoes rather than fried, as potato will absorb up to one third of its weight in fat. Mashed potato contains the least vitamin C. The tubers begin to lose their optimum vitamin C content from the time of lifting, so that stored and much travelled potatoes bought in supermarkets have up to 50% loss of nutrients.

Potato City Cleansing Mask for Dirt & Grease

Make 1 tbsp (15 ml) potato juice and add to 1 tbsp (15 ml) fuller's earth. Mix to a paste and apply to skin and allow to dry thoroughly. Remove residue crust with tepid water and splash with cold water. Dry and apply skin softening elderflower or tomato toner.

✳ See p.132.

Tomato Essence

Raw, puréed, in aspic, marinated or just pure juiced tomatoes are full of healthy goodness. In times of glut of ripe tomatoes, the most flavoursome and powerful tomato essence for cooking purposes, can be obtained by slicing a few pounds (or kilos) of tomatoes and hanging in a muslin bag above a bowl to drip overnight to collect the clear liquid. To intensify flavour of tomato dishes, add 1 tsp (5 ml) to 1 tbsp (15 ml) to recipes, especially where tomato purée is an ingredient.

✳ ✳ See p.132.

Healing Uses: Both tomatoes and potatoes are important to diet and nutrition. Raw tomatoes are high in carotenoids (ß-carotene) and potassium, as well as vitamins C, E, and minerals. Lycopene, the carotenoid pigment that changes tomatoes to red, lessens damage caused by free radicals. Potatoes are a useful source of vitamin C, potassium, starch and fibre. They supply the most common and often largest amount of daily vitamin C intake to people in potato-eating countries. Anti-inflammatory potato juice (mixed with equal parts of cabbage juice) is useful for healing external ulcers, ulcerated colitis and diverticulitis internally. Potatoes can also help balance sugar levels in diabetics.

Home Uses: Slices of raw tomato will cleanse clogged pores and greasy skin. Hanging bunches of dried tomato leaves discourage insects in the house. Tomatoes are cooling and aid digestion by assimilating fats, oils and fried foods. They are both a laxative and diuretic, and are fortifying. Raw sliced potato provides an immediate vitamin C–rich face cleanser by simply rubbing it over the skin. A wineglass of potato juice in the morning will relieve constipation.

Organic Tomato Insect Spray

Put 1 pt (½ lt) of organic tomato leaves in a container and pour over 2 pt (1 lt) of boiled water. Allow to steep for an hour or so before straining. Transfer to a spray-gun to eliminate any unwanted insects.

Tip: Collect leaves when denuding plants of leaves for setting trusses.

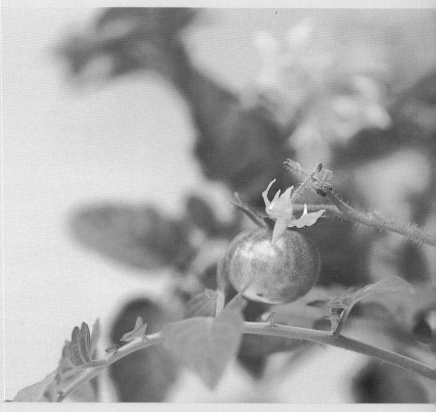

TOMATO (*LYCOPERSICON ESCULENTUM*)

Small Trees & Shrubs in a Tub

Small trees and shrubs express the largesse of the plant family in a convenient, portable manner. People can partake of their healing nature, either as a garden feature or as custodians to entrances, companionably sitting on front or back doorstep. Exotic plants in tubs have widespread appeal, from Mediterranean bay laurel; Oregon grape; the ornamental Japanese pepper, with its purple-red fruits, pungent bark and lemon-scented leaves; to the ancient Chinese *Ginkgo biloba*.

Small Trees & Shrubs in a Tub

Japanese Pepper (*Zanthoxylum piperitum*);
Bay Laurel (*Laurus nobilis*);
Maidenhair Tree (*Ginkgo biloba*);
Oregon Grape (*Mahonia aquifolium*)

Sweet Bay for Viral Infections

Use *Laurus nobilis* essential oil in massage (1 drop per 2 ml carrier oil) and/or (3-6 drops max.) in a bath. Alternatively, use leaves in bath-bag, or add leaf decoction (see p.123) to bath, and drink leaf infusion in small doses (see p.122) to alleviate colds and viral infections such as influenza, which affect appetite, causing dyspepsia, and aching muscles and limbs.
Cautions: A patch test is required for sensitivity in use of massage oil. Gardeners should take care that no other laurel is used in any medicinal way, as all are poisonous except *Laurus nobilis*.
Tip: Bay leaves added to flour, rice or dried pulses deters weevils. Fresh leaves incorporated with other herbs can be hung up to dry in the kitchen as a decorative culinary wreath.

✳ ✳ ✳ See p.132.

Liver & Gall Oregon Grape Jelly

Using the dried roots, clean and place 2 heaped tbsp (30 ml) in a pan with 1 pt (½ lt) of water. Cover, boil and simmer for 30 minutes to make a strong decoction. Cool and strain. Measure the strained liquid and for every pint made add agar-agar gelatine according to proprietary instructions. Return to heat, cool until liquid sets on a saucer. Pour into clean, dry, glass jar(s). Seal, label and date.
Tips: Any setting problems can be corrected with proprietary fruit pectin. To avoid the crown of the Oregon grape plant being eaten in hard weather (squirrels can be partial to it), protect the main stem with chicken-wire.

✳ See p.132.

Gentleman's Hair Oil

Add ½ tsp (2 ml) bay laurel and ¼ tsp (1 ml) lavender essential oils (3%) to 4 fl oz (100 ml) light coconut oil. Split into two 2 fl oz (50 ml) amber glass dropper bottles. Put few drops of oil on palm, sweep hairbrush over palm to absorb oil and brush into hair. Use circular movements to increase follicle circulation, bring dandruff to surface and allow oil to penetrate scalp. Leave for 30 mins before shampooing. Store oil in dark place.

Healing Uses: Japanese Pepper, *Hua jiao*, is a zingy, spicy, and carminative, scented ornamental herb. Its leaves, bark and seed container (pericarp) are an ancient stimulant for the spleen and stomach. Bay laurel aids digestion and is a stimulant and antiseptic. The root of *Mahonia aquifolium* promotes bile flow into the duodenum and is a bitter, astringent, liver tonic. *Ginkgo biloba*, derived from the Japanese *gin* meaning "silver" and *kyo*, "apricot" is used internally for asthma, allergies, and circulatory problems.
Home Uses: Used widely in flavourings in China, Hawaii and Japan, Japanese pepper's fruits have bactericidal and fungicidal properties, and its effects are best employed in culinary use as Thai "Five Spice" condiment, using leaves for soups and winter stews.

Sweet bay is a popular culinary herb and an infusion (see p.122) is good for digestion. A stimulating bath decoction (see p.123) will assuage tired limbs and focus the mind. Oregon grape jelly provides a simple culinary medicine for gall bladder complaints and diarrhoea. *Ginkgo biloba* leaves may be infused to help circulatory conditions such as varicose veins and Raynaud's disease.

Healing Ginkgo Biloba

This sacred tree of China and Japan evolved before mammals. It only fruits when conditions are clement, requiring separate male and female trees grown together. Originally found wild in provinces of Central China, it is conserved by cultivation and will happily start out in a tub for the patio, balcony or office windowsill. It can grow to be a great tree of immense girth, a fine specimen of which stands in the Physic Gardens, Chelsea, London.

Research into geriatrics' response has shown that the lignins and flavonoids contained in the leaves, actively improve cerebral function via circulation, carrying more oxygen to the brain. Thus gingko may be good for Alzheimers sufferers and may reduce the risk of stroke.

✳ See p.132.

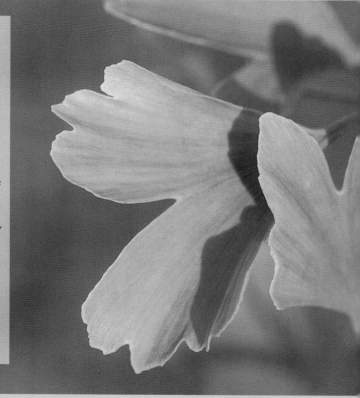

GINGKO (GINGKO BILOBA)

Soothing Herbal Patio Planter

Aloe brings a hint of the tropics into the micro-climate of a patio and looks particularly well placed in an urn. It will grow ready-to-hand for first-aid treatments in a more humble moveable clay pot in a window box in summer and on a kitchen windowsill in winter. Lemon verbena scents the air into late summer from sunshine and brick warmth if planted in any form of deep troughs against a wall. Its tall habit can be offset by planting it behind a rift of cleansing hyssop, which infusion is good for hay fever.

Soothing Herbal Patio Planter

Aloe (*Aloe vera*);
Hyssop (*Hyssopus officinalis*);
Lemon Verbena (*Aloysia triphylla*)

Maria Louisa in House & Garden

Alyosia triphylla (lemon verbena), named after Marie Louise (1791-1847), Empress of France, is commonly drunk as a mildly sedative and digestive "tea" throughout Spain and her territories. It has a lemony taste and aroma that is cleansing and bactericidal, relieving stomach spasms. A leaf decoction (see p.123) for cold compresses (see p.123) aids nausea and fever, and is reminiscent of *eau de verveine*, which was its famous perfume. A massage with the essential oil (2½ %, 1 drop per 2 ml) will help stomach cramps and liver congestion and alleviate anxiety, insomnia and nervous tension. Finely chopped leaves are good to flavour stuffings, add to summer drinks and salads, and for pot-pourris and herb pillows.
Tip: As in Victorian times, this is an ideal scented herb for conservatories.

Hyssop Infusions & Oil for the Body

This astringent and antiseptic biblical herb is strong and versatile. The green tops brewed as a "tea" will strengthen a weak stomach, whilst assisting muscular rheumatism or discoloured bruising. A leaf infusion (see p.122) "tea" is expectorant in action, and a "tea" of dried flowers will remedy a weak chest. An inhalation of hyssop essential oil helps asthma and bronchitis, and loosens catarrh. A massage (2½ %, 1 drop per 2 ml) helps to balance low or high blood pressure and assists the immune system against colds and influenza. It also allays fatigue and nervous tension, whilst aiding colic and indigestion that accompany colds and influenza.
Tip: Hyssop inhibits the growth of radishes, attracts bees and repels white cabbage butterflies.

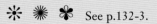 See p.132-3.

Aloe Vera for Hair

Add 1 tsp (5 ml) of aloe vera juice to 4 fl oz (100 ml) of base shampoo for light hair. Add 2½ % (1 drop per 4 ml each) of essential oils of invigorating rosemary and calming chamomile.

Healing Uses: A panacea for all ills, the healing properties of this ancient herb aloe, that Alexander the Great conquered the island of Socotra to secure, are fabled. An Ancient Egyptian remedy for digestive complaints, aloe sibaru, was prescribed by early Assyrian herbalists for the stomach and breathing difficulties. Aloe contains vitamins A, B_1, B_2, B_{12}, C and E; calcium, chromium, copper, magnesium, manganese, zinc, sodium chloride and potassium minerals; amino acids, enzymes, saponins, lignin, which can penetrate the skin, and anthraquinones, which are antibiotic, anti-viral, antibacterial and anti-inflammatory. It is particularly successful in relieving the symptoms of IBS.

Home Uses: Buy an aloe plant and keep it on the kitchen windowsill to have immediate access to the jelly contained in the leaves for burns and scalds. Aloe juice can be very successful in assisting colitis, kidney and liver ailments, and alleviating the pain of arthritis, and post-operative recovery. For minor digestive ailments use 1 tsp (5 ml) of aloe juice or jelly per day.

Hyssop flower tops made into a bath-bag make a purifying and healing ablution. Infused lemon verbena leaves can be used as a tonic "tea" and cleanser for cuts and abrasions. A decoction (see p.123) will provide an excellent sanitary floorwash for the sickroom.

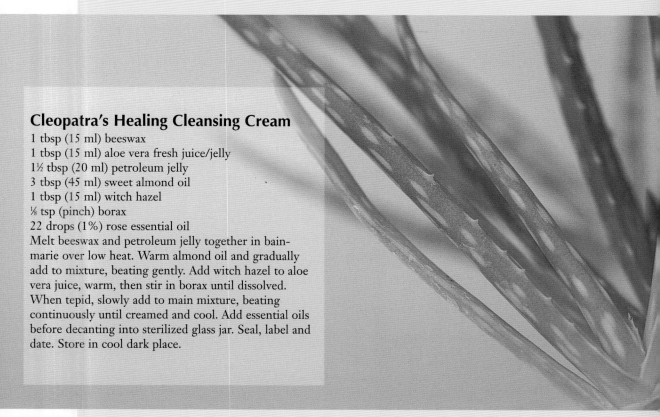

Cleopatra's Healing Cleansing Cream

1 tbsp (15 ml) beeswax
1 tbsp (15 ml) aloe vera fresh juice/jelly
1½ tbsp (20 ml) petroleum jelly
3 tbsp (45 ml) sweet almond oil
1 tbsp (15 ml) witch hazel
⅛ tsp (pinch) borax
22 drops (1%) rose essential oil

Melt beeswax and petroleum jelly together in bain-marie over low heat. Warm almond oil and gradually add to mixture, beating gently. Add witch hazel to aloe vera juice, warm, then stir in borax until dissolved. When tepid, slowly add to main mixture, beating continuously until creamed and cool. Add essential oils before decanting into sterilized glass jar. Seal, label and date. Store in cool dark place.

ALOE (ALOE VERA)

Summer Salad Hanging Basket

Basil is a holy and ancient herb universally native to warm climates. In a hanging basket, the spiritual colour of the "dark opal" *Ocimum basilicum* var. *purpurascens* is lifted skywards. Red orache, from Eastern Europe and Asia grows well in droughty or saline climates. The blazing bright peppery yellow and orange flowers of nasturtium form a fiery cascade, and together with rocket, a tangy Roman Mediterranean herb, common to Eastern Asia and North America, we have salad "lift off"!

Summer Salad Hanging Basket

Trailing nasturtiums (*Trapaeolum majus*);
Red Orache (*Atriplex hortensis* 'Rubra');
Purple Basil (*Ocimum basilicum* var. *purpurascens*);
Rocket (*Eruca vesicaria* subsp.)

Rocket

A digestive salad herb that has been used since the 1st century AD when it was recorded in *De Materia Medica*. It can be added at the last minute to stir-fries and pasta sauces. The whole plant is edible – flowers, seeds and oil.

Nasturtium Acne Cream

Recent trials in Germany by Dr Hauschka using antibiotic nasturtium for acne resulted in 83% improvement. The plant's ability to eliminate sulphur makes it highly suitable for this skin disorder in which sebaceous glands become inflamed. Acne is caused by overactivity of the glands in adolescence, usually on the face, chest and back, which can cause infected cysts and scarring of the skin. Dietary balance is essential. A nasturtium facial steam bath, followed by a double strength infusion (see p.122) as a wash and a decoction (see p.123) added to a base cream or lotion will produce good results.

Red Orache

Australian species *Atriplex nummularia* is a vegetable and can be employed to assist blood disease. Orache seeds have a similar effect to *Cephaelis ipecacuanha* and North American Indian *Gillenia trifoliata*, and are used professionally for amoebic dysentery and bronchial and asthmatic complaints respectively. Oraches are seldom eaten alone, but are good raw in mixed salads or used in cooking for colour with another vegetable like spinach. European common orache *A. patula* contains a high quantity of vitamin C.

Tip: Nip out the central shoot of orache to contain its upward growth.

Healing & Home Uses: Exotic basil is an important plant in Mexican herbalism and, after lotus (*Nelumbo nucifera*), the most sacred Indian herb in Ayurvedic medicine. *O. b.* var. *purpurascens*, pink flowering basil, is an ornamental, among which lemon basil (*O. b.* var. *citriodorum*) has a citrus twist. It is a good source of vitamins A and C and goes particularly well with tomatoes.

A restorative aromatic herb, basil is a natural tranquillizer. Leaf infusions (see p.122) relieve headaches associated with cold symptoms. It is effective against bacterial infections and intestinal parasites, and can be used as a tonic in wine or as an infusion for nausea and vomiting. A massage with French basil essential oil is analgesic, a nerve tonic, aiding muscular aches and pains, rheumatism, bronchitis and coughs. All fresh basils are useful for dyspepsia, stomach cramps, flatulence and nausea.

Red orache is a pot herb which stimulates metabolism, and eaten raw or cooked as a vegetable disperses sluggishness. Nasturtiums (see p.76) are antibiotic; the flowers are a cook's decorative delight, offering a welcome addition of vitamin C to the diet. Rocket leaves are a bitter and pungent tonic herb, excellent for digestion.

Sweet Basil for Nursing Mothers

Add 2 tsp (10 ml) sweet shredded basil to 1 cup boiling water. Cover and steep for 10 minutes, strain and drink. The infusion is a relaxant and will promote the increase of milk production in lactating mothers. It may be drunk three times a day over short periods.

Tip: Keep basil handy to rub bruised fresh leaves on bee stings to avoid swelling and reduce pain. Grow plants close to the house, as a fly repellent and keep a bunch in the house to absorb positive ions, energize negative ions and liberate ozone.

 See p.133.

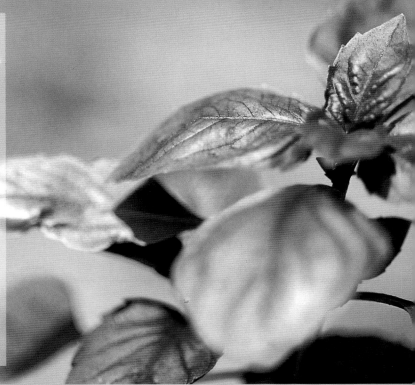

PURPLE BASIL (*OCIMUM BASILICUM VAR. PURPURASCENS*)

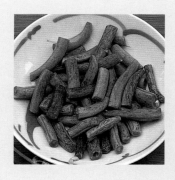

Chapter 8

Preparations

Gather herbs in dry weather, as soon as the dew has evaporated, to avoid humidity and subsequent mould. Remove any dead or damaged parts. Spread out to dry in a well-ventilated atmosphere. Small handfuls of culinary herbs for annual use can be successfully dried when bound at the stem, put into a brown-paper bag, tied in and hung upside down or placed in an airing cupboard.

Keep dried herbs in airtight jars, away from sunlight, whether home-dried or bought. The effectiveness of any herbal preparation is reliant on the quality of the herb and the strength of aroma. The smell and colour of the material is a good way to assess freshness when a collection date is not available.

TEAS AND INFUSIONS
Teas and simple infusions are alike. The plant material must not be boiled. Unless otherwise indicated, a basic "tea" or infusion of cut leaves, flowers and herbs requires: either 1 tsp (5 ml) dried herb, 2 tsp (10 ml) fresh herb (1 heaped) to 1 cup boiling water. Or 1 tbsp (15 ml) dried, 2 tbsp (30 ml) fresh herb (1 heaped) to 1 pint (½ lt) of boiling water. Cover and stand for 10 minutes, and strain before use. For washes etc, take a double handful of fresh herbs or

"Th'eclipse then vanishes and all her face
Is opened and restored to every grace;
The crust removed, her cheeks as smooth as silk
Are polished with a wash of asses' milk".
By Juvenal, Roman satirist (*c.* 60-140 AD)

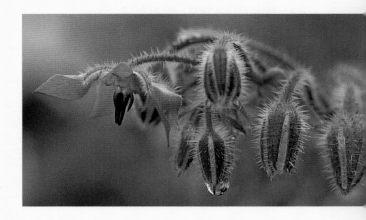

1oz (25-30g) and infuse for 30 minutes. Infusions stored in a refrigerator will last approximately 3 days.

Do not use aluminium, teflon or plastic containers. China and pyrex are best. Where applicable, strain the liquid into a jug before use. Preparations may be taken hot or cold. Hot infusions are sudorific and good for treating the common cold and influenza or in conditions where sweating is desired.

DECOCTIONS

Decoctions are used for bark, chips, roots and seeds, as well for producing stronger liquid for purposes other than drinking or where the remedy states such requirements. 1tbsp (15 ml) dried herb, 2 tbsp (30 ml) fresh herb to 1 pint (½ lt) of boiling water poured on to plant material, bring to the boil and simmer for 20-30 minutes, unless otherwise directed. Use containers as in "Teas" above. Due to reduction of liquid, it is necessary to add a little more water when decocting hard material such as berries. Refrigerate and use within a few days.

ESSENTIAL OILS

Essential oils are better bought – for safety and quality. The majority of plants are difficult to extract oils from and even minimal equipment is extremely expensive. Essential oils keep best in amber glass and must be stored in a cool dark place to protect them from photo-oxidation. Tops should never be left exposed to avoid oxidization. Keep essential oils out of the reach of children.

COMPRESSES

Use a clean cloth (linen, gauze or lint, padded with cotton wool) and soak in a hot decoction or infusion and apply as hot as possible (use an elbow test before applying). To keep in heat, cover with plastic. Re-apply as directed or necessary. Similarly, prepare and apply a cold compress from cold liquid, using refrigeration when essential. Some swellings require alternating hot and cold compresses.

Base Preparations

Lotions

For Dry Skin

**¼ pt (125 ml) floral water,
e.g. rosewater
¼ pt (125 ml) distilled witch hazel
5 drops glycerine**

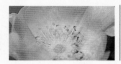

Blend the ingredients in a sterilized glass bottle and shake vigorously before use. Flower waters are gentle and softening, adding elasticity to the skin.

**4 tbsp (60 ml) dried plant material
4 tbsp (60 ml) ethyl alcohol
or 6 tbsp (90 ml) vodka
¼ tsp (1.25 ml) borax (a pinch)
3 tbsp (45 ml) distilled witch hazel
10 drops glycerine**

For Oily Skin

Macerate the plant material in alcohol for 14 days before straining. Dissolve the borax in the witch hazel and stir into the alcohol. Add in the glycerine and pour into a sterilized glass bottle. Shake well before use. Astringent herbs are most effective.

Syrup

Syrups "help the medicine go down", especially for children. A standard recipe is to add 1 1b (500 g) honey, or 12 oz (360 g) sugar to 1 pt (½ lt) of infusion or decoction. Warm, stirring until honey or sugar has dissolved and the mixture turns syrupy. Bottle, label, date and store in refrigerator.

Maceration

Macerated Oils

**3 tbsp (45 ml) herb
1 pt (½ lt) sweet almond oil
1 tbsp (15 ml) wine vinegar**

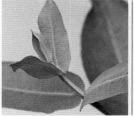

Put herbs and oil into a 2 pt (1 lt) container and add the vinegar. Close jar and place in sun, or in a very warm place in winter. Shake the jar each day. Allow to steep for 1 week, then strain and repeat process with current macerated oil three times or more. Strain, bottle in amber glass, label and date, and store in a dark cool place. Other forms of maceration employ cider vinegar or pure alcohol.

Ointments & Creams

Base Cream

2 tsp (10 ml) beeswax
1 tsp (5 ml) emulsifying wax
3 tsp (15 ml) almond/coconut oil
1 tsp (5 ml) avocado/nut kernel oil
4 tbsp (60 ml) double strength decoction
28 drops essential oils (95 ml)

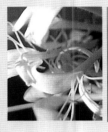

Melt the waxes in a bain-marie. Warm the oils and stir them in. Beat in the decoction and allow to cool before stirring in the essential oils. Decant into sterilized jars, seal, label and date. A drop of benzoin or myrrh (tincture or oil) will extend the life of a cream/ointment. Do not use borax on broken skin.

A boiled maceration in cold-pressed oil, like a strong decoction, makes a base herbal principle to add to ointments and creams. Essential oils added at 2½ % to petroleum jelly is another way to achieve a similar effect. Or 2½ % essential oil added to ready-prepared base creams and lotions, i.e. approx. 1 drop per 2 ml.

Poultice

Poultices are similar to compresses, except the moist plant material is used instead of the liquid alone. Mash or crush fresh plant material, either heating in a bain-marie or mix fresh or dried material with very little boiling water. Place between gauze, or two layers of cloth if the plant content is likely to cause irritation to the skin, and apply. Poultices retain their heat longer when mixed with bread, bran or other binding ingredients. They may be used to soothe aches and pains or withdraw toxins through the skin. It is a very good "on site" method of applying a plant's properties without deviation through the digestive tract.

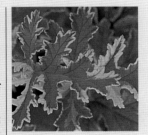

Powder

Many plants require bruising before maceration. Pulverizing a herb means to grind, bruise or mash the plant material with a pestle and mortar, or use an electric blender/grinder. For instance, rosehip shucks and culinary seeds may be treated in this way.

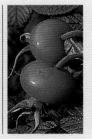

Recipes

Gardener's Nail Treatment

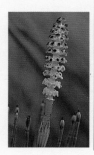

Use two adequately sized glass bowls to accommodate finger nails and toe nails. Keep in reserve 1 tbsp (15 ml) sweet almond oil (or sunflower/coconut oil). Put 2 tbsp (30 ml) chopped horsetail herb into stainless steel pan and pour over 1 cup boiled water. Cover and infuse for 20-30 minutes. Strain off horsetail plant material and pour into finger and toe bowls. Soak nails in liquid for 10-15 minutes. Remove, dry and massage almond oil into finger and toe nails. Store infusion in tightly closed glass container.

100 nettle stalks (with leaves)
2½ gal spring water (12 lt)
3 lb sugar (1½ kg)
2 oz cream of tartar (50 g)
½ oz yeast (15 g)

Nettle Beer Tonic

Clean nettles and boil in water for 15 minutes. Strain, add sugar and cream of tartar to liquid. Heat and stir until dissolved. Allow to become tepid, then add yeast and stir well. Cover with muslin and stand for 24 hours minimum. Best results are obtained if fermentation is allowed 4 days. Remove scum and decant without disturbing sediment. Bottle, cork and tie down.

(From *Wild Food* by Roger Phillips)

Pink Nerve Tonic Syrup

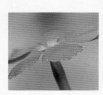

Pick and clean a sizeable double handful of prime carnation pink flower heads. Remove bitter white heels of petals, and place 1 oz (25 g) in heat-proof glass pouring jug. Pour over petals 1 fl oz boiling water, cover and allow to steep overnight or for half-a-day. Strain and add ½ lb (225 g) sugar, stirring continuously to dissolve. Bottle, label and date.

1-2 tsp (5-10 ml) fennel seeds
[1 tsp (5 ml) for children,
2 (10 ml) for adults]
1 cup boiling water

Slimming/Digestive Fennel Tea

An excellent tonic for the kidneys & liver.

Gently crush fennel seeds and add to boiling water. Cover and stand for 5-10 minutes. Drink 1 cup twice a day.

See p.132
See p.132

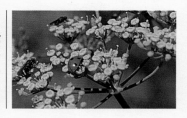

American Power Tea

1 tsp (5 ml) ginseng dried root
1 cup boiling water

For the stressed mind and body.

Grind 1 tsp (5 ml) ginseng dried root (in coffee grinder kept for this purpose), put in pot, and pour over 1 cup boiling water. Cover and stand for 15 minutes. Strain, if not enclosed in tea-infuser and sweeten with honey to taste. Ginseng is a great tonic for the whole body and an aphrodisiac.

❋ See p.132.
❋ See p.132.

Analgesic Migraine Brew

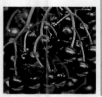

To be taken at first sign or onset of headache. Gather sprig of elderberries and wash clean. To 1 cup water add 10-15 berries. Mash mixture together. Place in pan, bring to boil and allow to simmer for 10 minutes. Strain through sieve. Sweeten with honey.

American Pumpkin Blossom Tea

3 pumpkin blooms
1 cup boiling water

This drink contains vitamins and minerals, and can be taken frequently as a tonic for the prostate gland.

Pick pumpkin blooms, place in jug and pour over boiling water. Cover and steep for 10 mins. Strain and sweeten to taste.

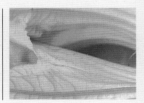

Deep-Pore Cleansing Plum Mask

Add half-handful oatmeal to half-handful sweet almonds. Pulverize in coffee grinder. To 2 tbsp (30 ml) of mixture, add pulp and juice of plums. Liquidize and apply to skin. If there are any lesions present add 1 tsp (5 ml) honey to help the healing process.

Astringent Plum Face Mask

6-7 plums
1 tbsp (15 ml) of spring water
1 tsp (5 ml) almond oil

Especially good for acne sufferers.

Boil plums with spring water. Allow to cool, extract kernels and mash insides of plums to pulp. Decant into liquidizer. Add almond oil and blend.

1 small handful cornflower blooms
1 cup boiling water
1-2 tsp (5-10 ml) honey

Cornflower Calming Tea

Said to be useful in helping recovery after a stroke, by aiding the return of motor abilities.

Take cornflower blooms and pour over boiling water. Cover and steep for 10 minutes. Strain and sweeten to taste with honey.

2 tsp (10 ml) beeswax
1 tsp (5 ml) emulsifying wax
3 tsp (15 ml) sweet almond oil
1 tsp (5 ml) avocado oil
10 drops each of rosemary, fennel, and juniper berry essential oils.

Hedera Massage Cream for Cellulite

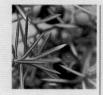

Make double strength ivy decoction with 4 tbsp (60 ml) ivy leaves to 1 pt (½ lt) water. Melt waxes in bain-marie. Warm oils and stir them in carefully. Beat in ivy decoction and allow to cool before adding essential oils. Decant into jar(s), close, label and date.

Place cucumber slices on tired or inflamed eyes or use as "mask" protection. Dice one-half cucumber and liquidize to paste for cold compress. For entire body treatment in cases where body-skin is inflamed overall, using at least a whole cucumber, liquidize into "juice" and gently apply, rather than massage, all over affected area. Useful to relieve sunburn and scalds.

Cooling Skin Inflammations

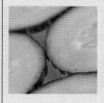

2 tsp (10 ml) beeswax
1 tsp (5 ml) apricot kernel oil
3 tbsp (45 ml) double strength lavender flower decoction (see p.123) or distilled lavender water
3 tsp (15 ml) sweet almond oil or lavender macerated oil, or else use 2 tsps (10 ml) sweet almond oil to 1 tsp (5 ml) rosehip oil
1 tsp (5 ml) emulsifying wax
40 drops pure essential lavender oil

Lavender Healing Cream

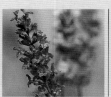

In bain-marie, melt waxes. Warm oils and stir them into waxes. Beat in decoction/lavender water and allow to cool before dropping and mixing in lavender essential oil. Put into glass jar(s), cover, seal, label and date. The use of vitamin C enriched rosehip oil will enhance healing quality.

Hypertension Tea

A remedy to aid obesity, heart, headache, stomach and blood.

Pick aromatic, bitter flowers of *Ju hua* (chrysanthemum) as required. Pluck and de-tail white heels of petals. Infuse 1 tsp (5 ml) prepared petals to 1 cup water. Cover and rest for 10-15 mins., according to taste.

Nourishing Carrot Eye Cream

1 tsp (5 ml) beeswax
3 tbsp (45 ml) rosewater
1 tsp (5 ml) lanolin
1 tbsp (15 ml) macerated carrot
½ tsp wheat germ oil
6 tsp (30 ml) each of sweet almond and coconut oil
15 drops carrot seed essential oil
¼ tsp (1¼ ml) borax

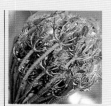

Suitable for use on all facial skin of mature complexions and for wrinkles.

Melt beeswax and lanolin together in bain-marie, stirring constantly. Warm oils and gradually beat them into waxes. Separately, dissolve borax in rosewater and slowly add to mixture, beating until cool. Gently stir in carrot seed oil as mixture thickens. With spatula, fill jars. Seal, date and label.

Lilac Zing Bath Bag

1 sizeable double handful of lilac flower heads
A few geranium leaves (2-3)

For a spring overall skin tonic.

Pick a sizeable double handful of lilac flower heads. Put the flowers into a muslin bag with a long string attached and add a few geranium leaves. Tie the bag to the bath tap and run water onto the contents. When in the bath, squeeze the bag periodically whilst soaking.

Balsam Bath Bag

A good cure for athletes, and the aged's aches and pains, and for nervous exhaustion.

Pick a double handful of young pine needles. Put needles in muslin bag tied with long string. Run hot bath. Bruise needles in bag with wooden mallet. Tie end of string to tap and lower into water. File nails or do other bodily chore to allow bath to lower in temperature, inhaling pine in the bathroom. Get into bath when temperature is comfortable and soak.

The following alternative may be more suitable for people with dry skin:

If aching, or suffering from a head cold, be indulgent. Use two bath bags, or add a strong pine needle decoction, and use pine needle ointment afterwards on affected areas. Alternatively, run a hot bath first and put in 3-6 drops maximum of pine essential oil just before getting into bath to soak and inhale.

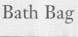
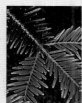

Conjunctivitis Eyebath Infusion

Take a small handful of cornflower blooms and pour on 1 cup of boiling water. Cover and steep for 30 minutes. Strain, and drink one cupful of "tea". Bottle remainder and use in eyebath.

Guelder Rose Concoction for Cramp

1-2 tbsp (15-30 ml) dried cramp-bark (Guelder Rose)
1 pt (½ lt) spring water

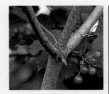

Use dried cramp-bark, stripped before autumn leaves change colour or leaf buds open in spring. Grind the dried bark in a coffee grinder (specially set aside for this purpose). Put ground dried herb in pot, pour over spring water and cover. Simmer for 20-30 minutes. Strain into jug. Apply warm directly to areas of cramp.

Celtic Corn Poultice

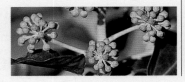

A useful poultice to draw boils, abscesses and carbuncles.

Take a double handful of ivy leaves, chop and boil in least possible water until tender. Place on affected site, bind and allow to "draw". Repeat until corn comes away with its root.

Egyptian Sprain Care for Hands and Feet

1 oz (25 g) chopped chervil plant (leaves & stems)
1 pt (½ lt) boiling water

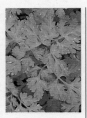

Treat sprain immediately with an infusion (see p.122). To prepare poultice, place chopped chervil plant (leaves and stems) crushed in large jug, and pour over boiling water. Cover and stand for 10-15 minutes. Strain liquid into small basin adequate to cover wrists or ankles (keeping aside plant material), and soak for 20 minutes. Take plant material and place between two layers of muslin, place on site of sprain and bind with bandage and rest. If knees are sore, use infusion to bathe and bind on poultice afterwards. Repeat treatment for 3 days, or longer, to help decoagulate any bruising under skin. Also drink the infusion as a "tea".

1 heaped tsp fresh sweet chestnut leaves
1 cup boiled spring water

Whooping Cough Control

Suitable for paroxysmal coughs with excess mucus.

Collect and shred fresh chestnut leaves immediately before infusing and pour over boiled spring water. Cover and stand for 10 minutes before drinking. If a cold infusion is needed, leave cup of mixture covered overnight to drink cold.

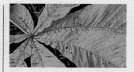

Anti-depressant Spring Primrose Infusion

3 tsp dried primrose flowers & leaves
2 cups (450 ml) boiling water

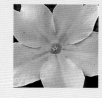

A suitable remedy for headaches and insomnia.

Place dried primrose flowers and leaves in heat-proof jug, and pour over boiling water. Cover and stand for 15 minutes. Strain and sweeten with honey to taste. Drink warm or hot throughout day, reheating as necessary.

A useful lymphatic cleanser for skin complaints and a good support remedy for chronic degenerative diseases such as cancer.

Red Clover Tea

Add 1 cup of boiling water to 2 tsp of fresh or 1 tsp of dried red clover flowers. Cover and stand for 10 minutes and strain before use.

3 garlic cloves finely chopped or crushed for immediate use
3-4 oz (90-125 g) fresh chopped basil leaves
4 fl oz (125 ml) extra virgin olive oil (enough to make thick paste)
sea salt
2 oz (60 g) freshly grated parmesan cheese (optional)
3-4 tbsp chopped pine kernels

Mediterranean Health Guard Pesto

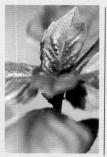

Traditionally the sauce of pastas, pesto incorporates a sound preventive medication in diet against heart disease and indigestion. Coriander can be interchanged with basil for a tonic.

Using mixer or liquidizer, purée garlic, adding basil to form pulp. Add oil and purée again until thick. Season with salt and add pine kernels (and parmesan if desired), mixing to thick paste. Store in glass jar, covering neck top with film of olive oil and refrigerate. This will keep for about 2 weeks or will freeze for up to 6 months.

Plant Cautions

✳ General warnings

Silver birch: Use fresh leaves, and not after midsummer.

Mountain ash: Rowan seeds are poisonous.

Juniper: The herb can interfere with the absorption of iron and minerals when taken internally.

Broom: Do not take internally except under medical supervision. Overdose can be fatal. Subject to legal restrictions in some countries.

Shrub roses, hips: Rosehip seed hairs irritate the digestion. Stew and sieve fruits before use.

Honeysuckle: The entire plant of the black (*Lonicera nigra*) and fly (*Lonicera xylosteum*) honeysuckle species are toxic. The seeds of all honeysuckle species are toxic.

Carrots: Excessive intake of carrot juice can cause skin discolouration and severe problems.

Alliums: Only add garlic to infused oils to be used within 3 days, as it attracts harmful bacteria.

Asparagus: High in purines; aggravates gouty conditions.

Comfrey: Toxic to the liver. It prevents iron absorption. Do not take internally at home.

Sage: Do not take in large doses.

Coriander: Use seed and essential oil in moderation.

Chickweed: Excess can cause diarrhoea and vomiting.

Horsetail: Not to be taken internally or by people over 55 years or for longer than 6 weeks without professional advice.

Ivy: Do not take internally.

Ginkgo biloba: Excessive use can cause dermatitis, headaches and vomiting.

Potatoes: Do not eat green or sprouting potatoes. They may cause drowsiness or migraine.

Tomatoes: Tomato's oxalic acid content is not good for kidney stones or acute rheumatism.

Bay laurel: Infusions in excess are emetic.

Hyssop: Use the essential oil in moderation.

Fennel: When taken internally interferes with iron and mineral absorption. Use the essential oil externally only.

Ginseng: Excess can cause high blood pressure and headaches. Do not take with caffeine or alcohol.

✳ Avoid in pregnancy

Juniper: Do not use in pregnancy or lactation.

Rosemary: Do not use in pregnancy or lactation.

Broom: Do not use in pregnancy or lactation.

Bergamot: Do not use the herb or oil in pregnancy.

Mint: Do not use pennyroyal herb or oil in pregnancy.

Lovage: Do not use if contemplating, or in, pregnancy.

Tarragon: Do not use the herb or oil in pregnancy.

Parsley: Do not use the seeds in pregnancy.

Sage: Do not use in pregnancy.

Thyme: Do not use in pregnancy.

Chickweed: Do not use in pregnancy.

Cowslip: Do not use in pregnancy.

Horsetail: Do not use if contemplating, or in, pregnancy.

Dandelion: Do not use if contemplating, or in, pregnancy or lactation.

Bay laurel: Do not use the oil in pregnancy.

Fennel: Do not use in pregnancy.

Ginseng: Do not use in pregnancy.

Oregon grape: Do not use the root in pregnancy.

✳ Avoid if allergic or skin sensitive

Silver birch: Do not use if sensitive to salicylates.

Juniper: If prone to allergies take a test patch before use.

Eucalyptus: Those prone to sensitization should not use the lemon-scented *E. citriodora*.

Rosemary: Except for creams, lotions and inhalations, the essential oil must be diluted.

Strawberries: Do not take if allergic to aspirin.

Nasturtium: Contains oxalic acid to which some people are allergic. In quantity it can be toxic.

Thyme: The oil can irritate the skin in some people. Always do a patch test before use.

Chickweed: Some people may be allergic to lanolin. Do a patch test before use.

Cowslip: Do not take if allergic to aspirin.

Dandelion: Avoid if allergic to gluten.

Tomatoes: Can trigger allergies, mouth ulcers and eczema in some people. For those prone to migraine, green tomatoes can trigger an attack.

Calendula: Some people may experience contact dermatitis. Do a test patch before use.

Bay laurel: Do not use if prone to dermatitis.

Hyssop: The essential oil may cause sensitization in some skin types; requires a patch test before use.

French basil: Essential oil may cause sensitization in some people. Do a test patch prior to use.

☼ Must be diagnosed/treated by professional medical doctor

Magnolia: Must not be used internally by non-professionals.

Hawthorn: Any serious heart disease must be treated by a medical practitioner.

Hollyhock/mallow: Gastric ulcers require diagnosis by a professional consultant.

Forget-me-not: Pleurisy requires professional supervision.

Poppy: Never use *Papaver somniferum* for home use.

Phlox: Bronchitis requires medical supervision.

Violet: Eczema requires professional diagnosis.

Carrots: Cancer must be diagnosed by a medical doctor.

Globe artichoke: Artichoke extract should only be used under professional supervision.

✳ Do not use for children
Blackthorn:
Should never be used for infants or children.

Honeysuckle: The berries can be fatal to children.

Mint: Do not use pennyroyal oil for young children.

Horsetail: Not suitable for young children.

Nettles: Do not feed to infants or young children.

❋ Contraindicated if you have specific complaint or are taking medication

Juniper: Do not use if you suffer from kidney complaints.

Rosemary: Avoid if suffering from high blood pressure, or epilepsy.

Broom: Avoid if you have high blood pressure, heart or kidney problems.

Blackthorn: Do not drink sloe liqueur if taking medication.

Hawthorn: Do not take if on prescribed medication.

Mint: Do not use pennyroyal oil in large doses if you suffer from kidney problems.

Parsley: Do not take seed or oil if you have kidney disease.

Cowslip: Do not take if using anticoagulant medication.

Hyssop: Do not use if epileptic.

Poisonous Plants List

Herbs vary in levels of toxicity, which can also depend upon use, whether eaten as food or administered in other modes internally. Some people may have a sensitive dermal disposition. Plants contain chemicals that are remedial, but in excess can poison. Everything on earth that can heal can also harm. Dosage is important to this balance, especially in the case of essential oils where it is advised a skin "patch test" is done before use and dosage not exceeded. Care should be taken with fresh and dried culinary herbs which contain small amounts of essential oils. It is not usually understood that when extracted the concentration of essential oils is far greater, even for external use.

Clematis (*Clematis* species)
Cowslip (*Primula veris*)
Daffodil & narcissus (*Narcissus pseudo narcissus* & *N. poeticus*)
Daphne (*Daphne* species)
Deadly nightshade (*Atropa bella-donna*)
Delphinium (*Delphinium* species)
Euphorbia (*Euphorbia* species)
Foxglove (*Digitalis* species)
Glory lily (*Gloriosa* species)
Lily of the valley (*Convallaria majalis*)
Madagascar periwinkle (*Catharanthus roseus*)
Meadow saffron (*Colchicum* species)
Monkshood (*Aconitum* species)
Opium poppy (*Papaver somniferum*)
Pokeroot (*Phytolacca* species)
Woody nightshade (*Solanum dulcamara* & *sp. varigatum*)

Glossary

Abortifacient: Inducing abortion or miscarriage.

Absolute: A highly concentrated, viscous, semi-solid or solid perfume material.

Adrenal glands: Two glands, covering the superior surface of each kidney.

Alkaloid: One of a diverse group of nitrogen-containing substances that are produced by plants and have potent effect on body function.

Allergen: Any antigen that causes allergy in a hypersensitive person.

Allergy: A disorder in which the body becomes hypersensitive to particular antigens which provide characteristic symptoms when encountered.

Alzheimers: A progressive form of dementia for which there is no cure.

Amenorrhoea: The absence or stopping of menstruation.

Amino acids: Fundamental constituents of all proteins. Essential amino acids are those that must be obtained from protein in the diet.

Analgesic: Relieving pain.

Anodyne: Soothes and eases pain.

Anorexia: Loss of appetite. Psychological state using starvation, vomiting and laxatives for weight loss.

Antibody: A blood protein that is synthesized in lymphoid tissue in response to a particular antigen and circulates in the plasma to attack the antigen and render it harmless.

Anti-coagulant: Prevents blood clots.

Antidote: Counteracts effects of poison.

Antigen: Any substance the body regards as foreign, or potentially dangerous, against which it produces an antibody.

Antihistamine: Used to treat allergic conditions.

Antisclerotic: Helps prevent the hardening of tissue.

Anti-seborrhoeic: An agent, relating to the skin, which helps control sebum production.

Aphrodisiac: Promotes sexual excitement.

Aromatherapy: The therapeutic use of essential oils in massage, etc.

Arteriosclerosis: Loss of elasticity in the artery walls due to thickening and calcification.

Astringent: Causing contraction of the tissues; binding.

Atheroma: Degeneration of the wall of the arteries due to the formation of fatty plaques and scar tissue, restricting blood circulation.

Aura: Medically, the forewarning of an attack. Spiritually, a subtle emanation attending a person or thing.

Bactericidal: Able to kill bacteria.

Bain-marie: Double saucepan: upper half for cooking sauces, lower half holds hot water.

Balsam: A resinous semi-solid mass or viscous liquid exuded from a plant.

Base oils: See fixed oils.

Bechic: Relieves coughs.

Blood lipid: A substance involved in the clotting of blood, important for the activation of plasma.

Blood platelet: A structure in blood relating to the arrest of bleeding.

Calmative: Produces a calming affect.

Cancer: A malignant tumour.

Carcinogen: Any substance that may cause the production of cancer.

Cardiac: Relating to the heart.

Carminative: Relieves flatulence.

Cathartic: Laxative or purgative, causing a violent purging of the body.

Cellulite: Accumulation of toxins due to an excess of fat in the tissue.

Cephalic: Of or relating to the head.

Cerebral: Pertaining to the largest part of the brain.

Chakra: A term given to an Indian system of energy centres of the body, roughly corresponding with the endocrine gland system.

Cholesterol: Fat-like material in blood and most tissues. Excess can cause gall stones.

Cirrhosis: A condition in which the liver responds to injury or death of some of its cells, becoming characteristically knobbly. Caused by alcoholism, hepatic viruses, etc.

Cicatrisant: Promotes healing by the formation of scar tissue.

CNS: Central nervous system.

Coagulate: Conversion of blood from liquid to a solid state.

Coeliac: Sensitivity to the protein gliadin contained in gluten.

Co-enzyme: A non-protein organic compound that in the presence of an enzyme plays an essential role in the reaction catalyzed by the enzyme.

Concrete: A concentrated, waxy, solid or semi-solid perfume material prepared from live plant matter.

Cystitis: Inflammation of the bladder, often caused by infection.

Demulcent: Substances which soothe and protect the alimentary canal.

Depressant: Reduces nervous or functional activity.

Dermatitis: Inflammation of the skin caused by an outside agent.

Diabetes: Any disorder of the metabolism causing excessive thirst and the production of large volumes of urine.

Diaphoretic: Promotes perspiration.

Diuretic: Increases the volume of urine produced by promoting excretion of salts and water from kidneys.

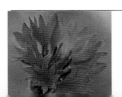

Dysmenorrhoea: Painful and difficult menstruation.

Dyspepsia: Disordered digestion.

Embolism: The condition in which an embolus becomes lodged in an artery and obstructs its blood flow.

Embolus: Material, such as blood clot, fat, air, or a foreign body, that is carried by the blood from one point in the circulation to lodge at another.

Emetic: Causes vomiting.

Emmenagogue: Stimulates menstruation.

Emollient: Soothes and softens skin.

Epilepsy: Any one of a group of disorders of brain function characterized by recurrent sudden attacks.

Essential oil: A volatile oil derived from an aromatic plant constituting the odorous principles of a plant.

Expectorant: Causes coughing; loosening of phlegm from chest and throat.

Fatigue: Inability of an organism, an organ, or a tissue to give a normal response to a stimulus until a certain recovery period has elapsed.

Febrifuge: Reducing fever.

Fixed oil: Vegetable oil obtained from plants which, distinct from essential oils, is fatty, dense and non-volatile, such as olive oil.

Flatulence: Having gases in the intestine; distension.

Flavonoids: Active plant constituents which improve circulation and can also have diuretic, anti-inflammatory and anti-spasmodic effects.

Fungicide: Prevents and kills fungi.

Gastritis: Inflammation of the stomach lining.

Gastroenteritis: Inflammation of the stomach and intestine, usually caused by viruses or bacteria.

Genito-urinary: Referring to both the genital and reproductive systems.

Gingivitis: Inflammation of the gums caused by plaque on the teeth, leading to swelling and easy bleeding.

Haemorrhoids (piles): Enlargement of the normal spongy blood-filled cushions in the wall of the anus.

Hepatic: Relating to the liver.

HRT: Hormone Replacement Therapy.

Hyperactivity: Abnormal increased activity.

Hypertension: High blood pressure.

Hypo: Below or less than normal.

IBS: Irritable Bowel Syndrome.

Immune system: The body's protective system which provides antibodies to defend against infection and disease.

Incontinence: Inappropriate involuntary passage of urine, resulting in wetting, or inability to control bowel movements.

Iodine: A trace element necessary to thyroid gland funtion.

Jaundice: Yellowing of skin and/or white of eyes, indicating excess bilirubin in the blood.

Lactation: The secretion of milk by the mammary glands of the breasts, beginning at the end of pregnancy.

Laxative: An agent used to stimulate bowel evacuation, or to encourage a softer or bulkier stool.

Lesion: A zone of tissue with impaired function as a result of damage by disease or wounding.

Leucocyte: White blood cells involved in protecting the body against foreign substances and in antibody production.

Leucorrhoea: A whitish or yellowish discharge from the vagina.

Limbic system: A complex system of nerve pathways and networks in the brain involved in the expression of instinct and mood in activities of the body's endocrine and motor systems.

Lumbar: Relating to the part of the body between the lowest ribs and the hip bones.

Lymph: The fluid present within the vessels of the lymphatic system.

Lymphatic system: A network of vessels that conveys electrolytes, water and proteins in the form of lymph, from the tissue fluids to the bloodstream.

Mastitis: Inflammation of the breast, usually caused by bacterial infection.

Menopause: Normal cessation of the menstrual cycle for women.

Menstrual cycle: The periodic sequence in sexually mature non-pregnant women whereby an egg cell is released from the ovary at four-weekly intervals until the menopause.

Micro: A prefix denoting small size or one-millionth part.

Mucilage: A substance containing gelatinous constituents which are demulcent.

Narcotic: Applied to substances producing stupor or insensibility.

Nephritis: Kidney inflammation.

Nervine: Strengthens and tones the nerves and the nervous system.

Neuralgia: A stabbing pain along a nerve pathway.

Oedema: Excessive accumulation of fluid in the body tissues.

Oestrogen: One of a group of steroid hormones that control female sexual development, growth and function.

Olfaction: The sense of smell and process of smelling.

Organic: Relating to any or all of the organs of the body or describing chemical compounds containing carbon, found in all living systems. Also, natural growth of plants without use of chemicals, pesticides, etc.

Osmosis: The passage of a solvent through a semi-permeable membrane, e.g. cell wall.

Osteoporosis: Loss of bone tissue resulting in bones that are brittle and liable to fracture.

Oxalic acid: Extremely poisonous acid, found in many plants including sorrel and rhubarb leaves. Antidote is milk.

Pantothenic acid: A water-soluble vitamin helping release of energy from food and proper function of adrenal glands.

Pathogen: Bacteria and other micro-organisms that parasitize an animal, plant or human, producing disease.

Pleurisy: Inflammation of the pleura – the membranes surrounding the lungs.

PMT/PMS: Pre-menstrual tension/ pre-menstrual syndrome.

Prostate gland: Male sex gland, below bladder.

Psyche: The mind or soul of a person.

Purgative: See laxative.

Relaxant: Relaxes tension and overactive nerves and tissues.

Resin: A natural or prepared product, e.g. exudations from trees (balsam).

Reticular activating system: Nerve pathways in the brain concerned with the level of consciousness – from the states of sleep, drowsiness, and relaxation to full alertness and attention.

Rubefacient: Causing reddening of the skin.

Rutin: A flavonol useful in treatment of high blood pressure, diabetes, salicylate and arsenic poisoning, and allergies.

Salve: A healing ointment or substance that soothes or consoles.

Sciatica: Pain felt down the back, outer side of the thigh, leg and foot.

Sedative: Causing sedation, reducing nervous excitement.

Serum: The fluid that separates from clotted blood or blood plasma.

Silica: A non-toxic element present in human muscle, bone, blood, as well as in quartz crystals.

Sinusitis: Inflammation of one or more sinuses in the facial bones that communicate with the nose, usually caused by infection.

Solarize: Medicinal use of sunshine by natural solar energy.

Soporific: Inducing drowsiness or sleep.

Spermatogenesis: Production of mature spermatozoa in the testis.

Stomachic: Eases stomach pain; stimulates stomach secretions.

Sudorific: Producing copious perspiration.

Tannins: Astringent active plant constituents which precipitate proteins.

Thrombophlebitis: Inflammation of the wall of a vein.

Thujone: A terpene which is antiseptic and carminative, but relatively toxic. Contraindicated in pregnancy.

Tincture: A liquid herbal extract made by macerating plant material in alcohol and water.

Unguent: An ointment, sometimes perfumed, medicinal or both.

Volatile oil: An often aromatic substance contained within plants, which when extracted is called an essential oil.

Vulnerary: Heals wounds.

Bibliography

Baker, Margaret, **Discovering the Folklore of Plants,** Shire Publications, 1969.

Bellamy, David and Pfister, Andrea, **World Medicine: Plants, Patients and People,** Blackwell, 1992.

Bown, Deni, **Encyclopaedia of Herbs and Their Uses,** Dorling Kindersley, 1995.

Bremness, Lesley, Contrib Ed, **Pocket Encyclopaedia of Herbs,** Dorling Kindersley, 1990.

Evans-Schultes, Richard and Hofmann, Albert, **Plants of the Gods,** Healing Arts Press, 1992.

Genders, Roy, **Scented Flora of the World**, Robert Hale, 1977.

Genders, Roy, **The Cottage Garden Year**, Croome Helm, 1986.

Grieves, Mrs. M., **A Modern Herbal,** Tiger Books Int., London, Revised Edition, 1992.

Griffin, Judy, **Mother Nature's Herbal,** Llewellyn, 1997.

Harmer, Juliet, **The Magic of Herbs and Flowers**, Macmillan, London, 1980.

Harvey, Clare G. and Cochrane, Amanda, **The Encyclopaedia of Flower Remedies,** Thorsons, 1995.

Hyne Jones, T. W., **Dictionary of the Bach Flower Remedies**, The C. W. Daniel Company Ltd., 1976.

Jarvis, D. C., **Folk Medicine: A Doctor's Life-time Study of Nature's Secrets,** Henry Holt & Co., 1958.

Lawless, Julia, **The Encyclopaedia of Essential Oils,** Element Books, 1992.

Lawless, Julia, **Lavender Oil**, Thorsons, 1994.

Levene, Peter, **Aphrodisiacs - Fact and Fiction,** Javelin Books, 1985.

Lipp, Frank J., **Herbalism,** Macmillan ass. Duncan Baird Publishers, 1996.

Mabey, Richard, with Michael McIntyre, Gail Duff, John Stevens, **The Complete New Herbal**, Elmtree Books, 1988.

Manniche, Lise, **An Ancient Egyptian Herbal**, British Museum Press, 1989.

Meadows, Kenneth, **Earth Medicine**, Element Books, 1989.

Paterson, Jacqueline Memory, **Tree Wisdom**, Thorsons, 1996.

Peterson, Nicola, **Herbal Remedies**, Blitz Editions, 1995.

Petulengro, Leon, **Herbs and Astrology**, Darton, Longman & Todd Ltd, 1977.

Reader's Digest Association Ltd., **Foods that Harm, Foods that Heal,** 1996.

Reader's Digest Association Ltd, **1001 Hints and Tips for the Garden**, 1996.

Rose, Jeanne, **Kitchen Cosmetics**, North Atlantic Books, 1990.

Thomson, William, A. R., **Healing Plants - A Modern Herbal**, Macmillan London, 1980.

Williams, Jude C., **Jude's Herbal Home Remedies**, Llewellyn, 1994.

Winter Griffith, Dr. H., **The Vital Vitamin Fact File**, Thorsons, 1988.

Wren, R.C., **Potter's New Cyclopaedia of Botanical Drugs & Preparations**, The C. W. Daniel Co Ltd., (1907), 1985 update.

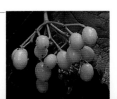

Subject Index

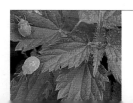

RECIPES AND PREPARATIONS

Plant Name Index

Acknowledgements

Author's Acknowledgements

I would like to express my thanks to the Ancients for first discovering that "for every disease there is in nature a severall symple". I am grateful to the generations of ordinary people who handed down their know-ledge, recipes and remedies to their successors. In my case I owe a special debt from early childhood to one such lady I called Grannie Woodland, and to many others along life's way. These heirs to natural medicine have kept alive the art of herbalism and made possible the prolific works of practitioners and authors that once more abounds and is referred to in the bibliography. My gratitude goes to the ever-patient and helpful librarians of The Royal Horticultural Society and Swiss Cottage reference library, the British Library and Aldwych Science Reading Rooms.

Publisher's Acknowledgements

Gaia Books would like to thank Deni Bown, the photographer for her tremen-dous contribution to this book, and for her resourcefulness. In addition we would like to thank her for checking the Latin plant names for accuracy. We would also like to thank Mary Warren, the proof-reader and indexer; Christine Steward, the Consultant Herbalist for checking the text for technical accuracy, and Sara Mathews for design direction.

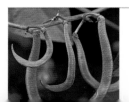

OTHER TITLES PUBLISHED BY GAIA BOOKS

HERITAGE VEGETABLES

SUE STICKLAND

£14.99

ISBN 1 85675 033 7

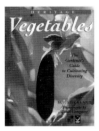

How to save and exchange the seeds of the most delicious and nutritious vegetables from our past. Advice on cultivation of varieties recommended for their suitability for specific soils and aspects.

HERBS FOR COMMON AILMENTS

ANNE MCINTYRE

£8.99

ISBN 1 85675 055 8

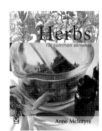

Reliable, traditional knowledge in a modern context. It explains the basics of herbalism and how to prepare your own herbs for safe treatments, self help, prevention and cure.

COMPLETE WOMAN'S HERBAL

ANNE MCINTYRE

£15.00

ISBN 1 85675 012 4

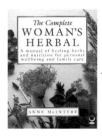

Healing herbs and nutrition for the cycles of a woman's life and for the family. A manual of holistic healthcare.

COMPLETE FLORAL HEALER

ANNE MCINTYRE

£15.99

ISBN 1 85675 067 1

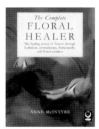

Rediscover the healing power of flowers for physical and emotional problems in this beautifully illustrated, authoritative manual.

SIMPLE HOME REMEDIES FOR COMMON AILMENTS

ANNE MCINTYRE

£8.99

ISBN 1 85675 086 8

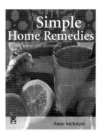

Successful and reliable cures for nearly 300 conditions. An invaluable resource for self help, prevention and first aid from your larder, bathroom cabinet and hedgerow.

To request a full catalogue of titles published by Gaia Books please call 01453 752985, fax 01453 752987 or write to Gaia Books Ltd., 20 High Street, Stroud, Gloucestershire, GL5 1AS e-mail address gaiabook@star.co.uk Internet address http://www.gaiabooks.co.uk